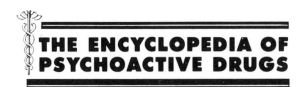

THE ENCYCLOPEDIA OF PSYCHOACTIVE DRUGS

SERIES 1

The Addictive Personality
Alcohol and Alcoholism
Alcohol Customs and Rituals
Alcohol Teenage Drinking
Amphetamines Danger in the Fast Lane
Barbiturates Sleeping Potion or Intoxicant?
Caffeine The Most Popular Stimulant
Cocaine A New Epidemic
Escape from Anxiety and Stress
Flowering Plants Magic in Bloom
Getting Help Treatments for Drug Abuse
Heroin The Street Narcotic
Inhalants The Toxic Fumes

LSD Visions or Nightmares?
Marijuana Its Effects on Mind & Body
Methadone Treatment for Addiction
Mushrooms Psychedelic Fungi
Nicotine An Old-Fashioned Addiction
Over-The-Counter Drugs Harmless or Hazardous?
PCP The Dangerous Angel
Prescription Narcotics The Addictive Painkillers
Quaaludes The Quest for Oblivion
Teenage Depression and Drugs
Treating Mental Illness
Valium The Tranquil Trap

SERIES 2

Bad Trips
Brain Function
Case Histories
Celebrity Drug Use
Designer Drugs
The Downside of Drugs
Drinking, Driving, and Drugs
Drugs and Civilization
Drugs and Crime
Drugs and Diet
Drugs and Disease
Drugs and Emotion
Drugs and Pain
Drugs and Perception
Drugs and Pregnancy
Drugs and Sexual Behavior

Drugs and Sleep
Drugs and Sports
Drugs and the Arts
Drugs and the Brain
Drugs and the Family
Drugs and the Law
Drugs and Women
Drugs of the Future
Drugs Through the Ages
Drug Use Around the World
Legalization A Debate
Mental Disturbances
Nutrition and the Brain
The Origins and Sources of Drugs
Substance Abuse Prevention and Cures
Who Uses Drugs?

DRUGS
&
PAIN

GENERAL EDITOR
Professor Solomon H. Snyder, M.D.

*Distinguished Service Professor of
Neuroscience, Pharmacology, and Psychiatry at
The Johns Hopkins University School of Medicine*

•

ASSOCIATE EDITOR
Professor Barry L. Jacobs, Ph.D.

*Program in Neuroscience, Department of Psychology,
Princeton University*

•

SENIOR EDITORIAL CONSULTANT
Joann Rodgers

*Deputy Director, Office of Public Affairs at
The Johns Hopkins Medical Institutions*

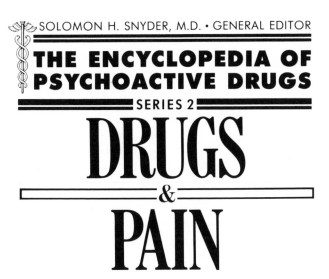

SOLOMON H. SNYDER, M.D. • GENERAL EDITOR

THE ENCYCLOPEDIA OF PSYCHOACTIVE DRUGS

SERIES 2

DRUGS & PAIN

JOANN ELLISON RODGERS

CHELSEA HOUSE PUBLISHERS
NEW YORK • NEW HAVEN • PHILADELPHIA

EDITOR-IN-CHIEF: Nancy Toff
EXECUTIVE EDITOR: Remmel T. Nunn
MANAGING EDITOR: Karyn Gullen Browne
COPY CHIEF: Perry Scott King
ART DIRECTOR: Giannella Garrett
PICTURE EDITOR: Elizabeth Terhune

STAFF FOR DRUGS AND PAIN:

SENIOR EDITOR: Jane Larkin Crain
ASSOCIATE EDITOR: Paula Edelson
ASSISTANT EDITOR: Michele A. Merens
DESIGNER: Victoria Tomaselli
COPY EDITORS: Sean Dolan, Gillian Bucky, Ellen Scordato
CAPTIONS: Louise Bloomfield
PICTURE RESEARCH: Emily Miller, Karen Herman
PRODUCTION COORDINATOR: Alma Rodriguez

CREATIVE DIRECTOR: Harold Steinberg

COVER: Egon Schiele, *Nudo Virile Con Drappo Rosso.* Art Resource.

Library of Congress Cataloging-in-Publication Data

Rodgers, Joann Ellison.
   Drugs & pain.
   (The Encyclopedia of psychoactive drugs. Series 2)
   Bibliography: p.
   Includes index.
   Summary: An examination of the origins and different
types of pain in the body and a discussion of the various
drugs and treatments that are available for pain relief.
   1. Pain—Juvenile literature. 2. Analgesia—Juvenile
literature. 3. Analgesics—Juvenile literature. [1. Pain.
2. Analgesia. 3. Analgesics] I. Title. II. Title: Drugs and pain.
III. Series.
RB127.R63   1987   615'.783   87-747

ISBN 1-55546-212-X

CONTENTS

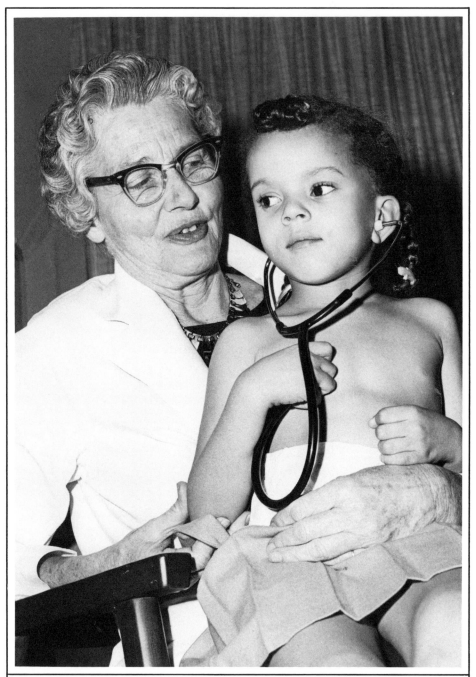

Many factors can affect the quest for freedom from pain. An empathic relationship between doctor and patient makes the sufferer a partner in his or her own treatment and sometimes hastens recovery.

FOREWORD

In the Mainstream
of American Life

One of the legacies of the social upheaval of the 1960s is that psychoactive drugs have become part of the mainstream of American life. Schools, homes, and communities cannot be "drug proofed." There is a demand for drugs — and the supply is plentiful. Social norms have changed and drugs are not only available—they are everywhere.

But where efforts to curtail the supply of drugs and outlaw their use have had tragically limited effects on demand, it may be that education has begun to stem the rising tide of drug abuse among young people and adults alike.

Over the past 25 years, as drugs have become an increasingly routine facet of contemporary life, a great many teenagers have adopted the notion that drug taking was somehow a right or a privilege or a necessity. They have done so, however, without understanding the consequences of drug use during the crucial years of adolescence.

The teenage years are few in the total life cycle, but critical in the maturation process. During these years adolescents face the difficult tasks of discovering their identity, clarifying their sexual roles, asserting their independence, learning to cope with authority, and searching for goals that will give their lives meaning.

Drugs rob adolescents of precious time, stamina, and health. They interrupt critical learning processes, sometimes forever. Teenagers who use drugs are likely to withdraw increasingly into themselves, to "cop out" at just the time when they most need to reach out and experience the world.

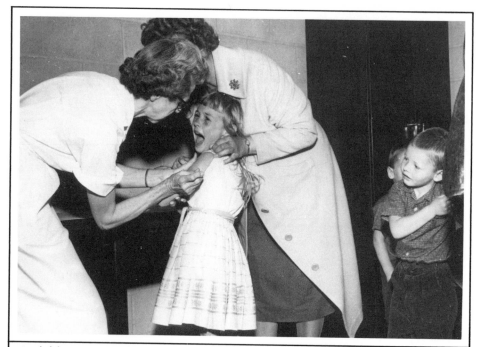

A child protests after receiving a shot. The realization that not all pain is bad or avoidable is an important part of growing up.

Fortunately, as a recent Gallup poll shows, young people are beginning to realize this, too. They themselves label drugs their most important problem. In the last few years, moreover, the climate of tolerance and ignorance surrounding drugs has been changing.

Adolescents as well as adults are becoming aware of mounting evidence that every race, ethnic group, and class is vulnerable to drug dependency.

Recent publicity about the cost and failure of drug rehabilitation efforts; dangerous drug use among pilots, air traffic controllers, star athletes, and Hollywood celebrities; and drug-related accidents, suicides, and violent crime have focused the public's attention on the need to wage an all-out war on drug abuse before it seriously undermines the fabric of society itself.

The anti-drug message is getting stronger and there is evidence that the message is beginning to get through to adults and teenagers alike.

The Encyclopedia of Psychoactive Drugs hopes to play a part in the national campaign now underway to educate young people about drugs. Series 1 provides clear and comprehensive discussions of common psychoactive substances, outlines their psychological and physiological effects on the mind and body, explains how they "hook" the user, and separates fact from myth in the complex issue of drug abuse.

Whereas Series 1 focuses on specific drugs, such as nicotine or cocaine, Series 2 confronts a broad range of both social and physiological phenomena. Each volume addresses the ramifications of drug use and abuse on some aspect of human experience: social, familial, cultural, historical, and physical. Separate volumes explore questions about the effects of drugs on brain chemistry and unborn children; the use and abuse of painkillers; the relationship between drugs and sexual behavior, sports, and the arts; drugs and disease; the role of drugs in history; and the sophisticated drugs now being developed in the laboratory that will profoundly change the future.

Each book in the series is fully illustrated and is tailored to the needs and interests of young readers. The more adolescents know about drugs and their role in society, the less likely they are to misuse them.

Joann Rodgers
Senior Editorial Consultant

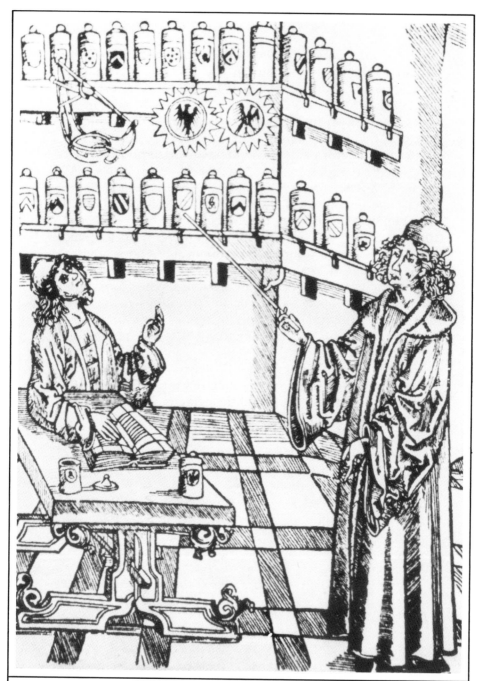

A 15th-century pharmacy, stocked with remedies the pharmacist himself prepared. In medieval Europe, witchcraft, superstition, and medical practices all played a role in the treatment of sickness or injury.

The Gift of Wizardry
Use and Abuse

JACK H. MENDELSON, M.D.
NANCY K. MELLO, Ph.D.

Alcohol and Drug Abuse Research Center
Harvard Medical School—McLean Hospital

Dorothy to the Wizard:

"I think you are a very bad man," said Dorothy.
"Oh no, my dear; I'm really a very good man; but I'm a very bad Wizard."
—from THE WIZARD OF OZ

Man is endowed with the gift of wizardry, a talent for discovery and invention. The discovery and invention of substances that change the way we feel and behave are among man's special accomplishments, and, like so many other products of our wizardry, these substances have the capacity to harm as well as to help. Psychoactive drugs can cause profound changes in the chemistry of the brain and other vital organs, and although their legitimate use can relieve pain and cure disease, their abuse leads in a tragic number of cases to destruction.

Consider alcohol — available to all and yet regarded with intense ambivalence from biblical times to the present day. The use of alcoholic beverages dates back to our earliest ancestors. Alcohol use and misuse became associated with the worship of gods and demons. One of the most powerful Greek gods was Dionysus, lord of fruitfulness and god of wine. The Romans adopted Dionysus but changed his name to Bacchus. Festivals and holidays associated with Bacchus celebrated the harvest and the origins of life. Time has blurred the images of the Bacchanalian festival, but the theme of drunkenness as a major part of celebration has survived the pagan gods and remains a familiar part of modern society. The term "Bacchanalian Festival" conveys a more appealing image than "drunken orgy" or "pot party," but whatever the label, drinking alcohol is a form of drug use that results in addiction for millions.

The fact that many millions of other people can use alcohol in moderation does not mitigate the toll this drug takes on society as a whole. According to reliable estimates, one out of every ten Americans develops a serious alcohol-related problem sometime in his or her lifetime. In addition, automobile accidents caused by drunken drivers claim the lives of tens of thousands every year. Many of the victims are gifted young people, just starting out in adult life. Hospital emergency rooms abound with patients seeking help for alcohol-related injuries.

Who is to blame? Can we blame the many manufacturers who produce such an amazing variety of alcoholic beverages? Should we blame the educators who fail to explain the perils of intoxication, or so exaggerate the dangers of drinking that no one could possibly believe them? Are friends to blame — those peers who urge others to "drink more and faster," or the macho types who stress the importance of being able to "hold your liquor"? Casting blame, however, is hardly constructive, and pointing the finger is a fruitless way to deal with the problem. Alcoholism and drug abuse have few culprits but many victims. Accountability begins with each of us, every time we choose to use or misuse an intoxicating substance.

It is ironic that some of man's earliest medicines, derived from natural plant products, are used today to poison and to intoxicate. Relief from pain and suffering is one of society's many continuing goals. Over 3,000 years ago, the Therapeutic Papyrus of Thebes, one of our earliest written records, gave instructions for the use of opium in the treatment of pain. Opium, in the form of its major derivative, morphine, and similar compounds, such as heroin, have also been used by many to induce changes in mood and feeling. Another example of man's misuse of a natural substance is the coca leaf, which for centuries was used by the Indians of Peru to reduce fatigue and hunger. Its modern derivative, cocaine, has important medical use as a local anesthetic. Unfortunately, its increasing abuse in the 1980s clearly has reached epidemic proportions.

The purpose of this series is to explore in depth the psychological and behavioral effects that psychoactive drugs have on the individual, and also, to investigate the ways in which drug use influences the legal, economic, cultural, and even moral aspects of societies. The information presented here (and in other books in this series) is based on many clinical and laboratory studies and other observations by people from diverse walks of life.

Over the centuries, novelists, poets, and dramatists have provided us with many insights into the sometimes seductive but ultimately problematic aspects of alcohol and drug use. Physicians, lawyers, biologists, psychologists, and social scientists have contributed to a better understanding of the causes and consequences of using these substances. The authors in this series have attempted to gather and condense all the latest information about drug use and abuse. They have also described the sometimes wide gaps in our knowledge and have suggested some new ways to answer many difficult questions.

One such question, for example, is how do alcohol and drug problems get started? And what is the best way to treat them when they do? Not too many years ago, alcoholics and drug abusers were regarded as evil, immoral, or both. It is now recognized that these persons suffer from very complicated diseases involving deep psychological and social problems. To understand how the disease begins and progresses, it is necessary to understand the nature of the substance, the behavior of addicts, and the characteristics of the society or culture in which they live.

Although many of the social environments we live in are very similar, some of the most subtle differences can strongly influence our thinking and behavior. Where we live, go to school and work, whom we discuss things with — all influence our opinions about drug use and misuse. Yet we also share certain commonly accepted beliefs that outweigh any differences in our attitudes. The authors in this series have tried to identify and discuss the central, most crucial issues concerning drug use and misuse.

Despite the increasing sophistication of the chemical substances we create in the laboratory, we have a long way to go in our efforts to make these powerful drugs work for us rather than against us.

The volumes in this series address a wide range of timely questions. What influence has drug use had on the arts? Why do so many of today's celebrities and star athletes use drugs, and what is being done to solve this problem? What is the relationship between drugs and crime? What is the physiological basis for the power drugs can hold over us? These are but a few of the issues explored in this far-ranging series.

Educating people about the dangers of drugs can go a long way towards minimizing the desperate consequences of substance abuse for individuals and society as a whole. Luckily, human beings have the resources to solve even the most serious problems that beset them, once they make the commitment to do so. As one keen and sensitive observer, Dr. Lewis Thomas, has said,

> There is nothing at all absurd about the human condition. We matter. It seems to me a good guess, hazarded by a good many people who have thought about it, that we may be engaged in the formation of something like a mind for the life of this planet. If this is so, we are still at the most primitive stage, still fumbling with language and thinking, but infinitely capacitated for the future. Looked at this way, it is remarkable that we've come as far as we have in so short a period, really no time at all as geologists measure time. We are the newest, youngest, and the brightest thing around.

DRUGS
&
PAIN

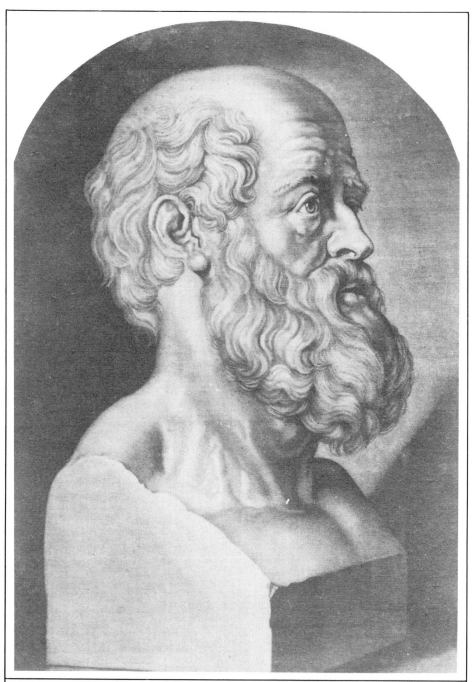

The ancient Greek physician Hippocrates devised a code of medical ethics that is still observed. Throughout history, the desire to ease pain has been a driving force among all health care professionals.

AUTHOR'S PREFACE

Because nothing holds our attention so fast and hard as physical pain, vast amounts of time, energy, and resources have been spent throughout history trying to stop or prevent it. Thomas Jefferson hit the mark when he wrote, "The art of life is the avoiding of pain."

In the 1980s avoiding pain is a serious industry. Americans spend $700 million a year on aspirin and similar products alone. In the past 150 years chemical pain relief has become a vast commercial success thanks to modern chemistry, the Industrial Revolution's assembly line, and the discovery of anesthetic gases.

The idea of using substances for pain relief has been a thriving enterprise for much longer than the last 150 years. Paleontologists have evidence of the prehistoric use of herbs and drugs to deaden pain. Sumerian scrolls describe the use of alcohol and opiates for pain in the Middle East in 4000 B.C.E. (B.C.E. or before the common era is the same as B.C.), and ancient Greek and Roman physicians used products from the opium poppy to treat migraine headaches, kidney stones, and cancer.

In the Andes mountains of South America, the Incas were well acquainted with the coca plant and its pain-numbing properties centuries before cocaine, derived from the plant, became a mainstream substance of abuse. Indeed, coca leaves were considered a divine gift by the Incas, whose holy men used them during ceremonial rites. Modern anesthesiologists like to point out that Genesis 2:21 — in which the Lord "caused a deep sleep to fall upon Adam, and he slept" before the "operation" to remove one of his ribs — suggests ancient knowledge, if not divine origins, of anesthesia.

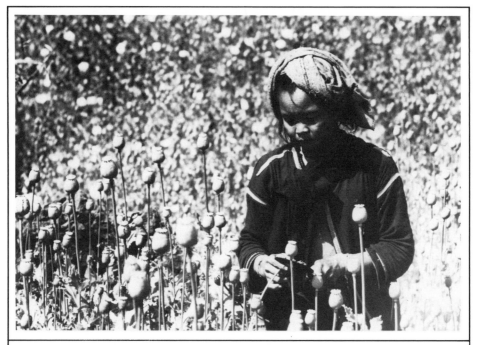

A Thai tribal woman harvests poppies, the source of heroin and opium. Opium was first used for pain relief in the Middle East as early as the 4th millennium B.C.E.

The reason pain and its conquest draw so much attention is no mystery. Pain is a universally shared — and exquisitely complicated — electrochemical event that accurately warns people against serious or lethal injury. From the instant of birth, people begin to look for, collect, refine, remember, and pass on ways to soothe their way through life. The process is as inevitable as a little girl's instinctive thrust of a pinched or burned finger into her mouth. By the time that child is grown she will have a knowledge of pain so personal, complicated, and subtle that she can choose from among 114 separate words in the English language alone to describe it.

The Most Common Symptom

According to the National Institutes of Health, pain is the most common medical symptom — as no doubt it was for our ancestors — and three or four kinds are experienced by most people each year. According to a recent survey conducted by Louis Harris and Associates for Bristol-Myers, 73% of

Americans 18 years of age and older suffer one or more headaches a year, 56% a backache, 46% stomach pains, 40% (of women surveyed) menstrual cramps, and 27% dental pain.

The survey also confirmed that younger people are far more likely than older people to experience headaches, backaches, muscle pains, stomach pains, menstrual cramps, and dental pains.

Overall, the survey determined that older teens and adults spent 23 days each year in too much pain to go about their normal routines. Although younger teenagers may heal faster, complain less, or cope better with some pain, they suffer no less. Adolescents suffer from headaches, menstrual cramps, muscle pulls, cuts, bruises, and writer's cramp as a result of their age, growth curve, school activities, and sports interests. They hurt from flu, fever, constipation, arthritis, impacted wisdom teeth, orthodontic work, inflammations, sprains, low-back trouble, tennis elbow, torn knee ligaments, and garden-variety "growing pains."

The prevalence of pain is the reason that the search for pain relief has attracted so much attention; likewise, the successes of modern chemistry and medicine explain the proliferation of proven painkillers available for the war against pain.

The latest edition of the *Physicians' Desk Reference*, a comprehensive catalog of brand-name prescription and non-prescription drugs approved for sale in the United States, lists more than 165 separate analgesic and narcotic drugs sold in an enormous variety of products. The U.S. Food and Drug Administration reports that more than 50,000 products containing aspirin are available to consumers.

There are almost 80 different general and topical anesthetics available in hundreds of separate products. Thousands of remedies are on sale for stomach pain, arthritis, infections, burns, inflammations, nausea, muscle cramps, heart disease, coughs, sinus congestion, and skin diseases. Americans swallow, gulp, inject, drink, and apply enough substances to support the now-famous observation by Sir William Osler — the renowned turn-of-the-century Canadian physician, researcher, and teacher — that "a desire to take medicine is, perhaps, the great feature which distinguishes man from other animals."

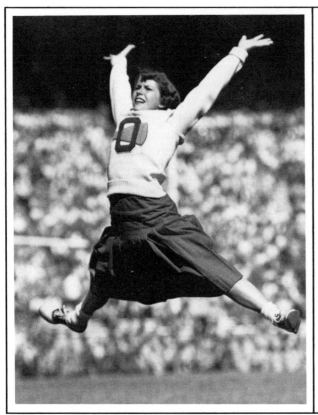

Cheerleaders may sustain painful injuries while engaged in calisthenics but may not feel the sensations until afterwards. Many teenagers do get hurt in the course of normal athletic activity, but fortunately, many of these "minor" injuries heal quickly and without complications.

Mixed Messages

No wonder, then, that most teenagers get mixed messages about drugs and their ability to combat physical pain. From the speedy-relief promises of television commercials to the home medicine chests crammed with prescription narcotics, teens encounter widespread acceptance of legal drugs that can stop or dull pain, and they are encouraged to use them. Unfortunately, teenagers are likely — as many adults are — to be overwhelmed and misled by the wide variety of conflicting advertising claims for painkilling drugs. They may also be unaware of side effects and potentially dangerous interactions of certain medications.

In addition, some teens are understandably puzzled — and even injured — by society's confused beliefs about pain. There are people, for example, who have mistaken ideas about the origin of pain and believe that pain is a punishment for some sin, that acceptance of pain is a mark of strong character, and that seeking pain relief is a sign of weakness.

In the past, physicians and theologians debated the use of anesthesia in childbirth, citing the biblical warning, "In sorrow thou shalt bring forth children." Some believed pain-less birth was immoral and threatened women's virtue. Some contemporary "philosophers" are no less provocative about the role of pain and its relief, as illustrated by the "no pain, no gain" pronouncements of athletic coaches and various exercise gurus.

The widespread use of illegal and dangerous drugs among teenagers has also led some adults — and teenagers — to resist the appropriate use of painkillers on the theory that "getting in the habit" of taking drugs — even for a good reason — is enough to get a person in the habit of taking drugs for not-so-good reasons.

Pain Relief

Intense interest in pain and its alleviation is one of the hall-marks of civilization, but meeting that interest safely and effectively is as tricky in the 1980s as it was millennia ago. This book is designed to help young people and all those who care about them navigate the tricky parts.

In this book they will learn what pain is and where it comes from; why some people seem to hurt more than others; how to assess pain; how classes of painkillers differ; how painkillers have their effects in the brain and the central nervous system; how the search for the perfect, nonaddictive analgesic is progressing; why pain is an ally in keeping fit and healthy; how pain is measured; what the worst kinds of pain are; how pain relief can be gained through nonchemical means; what the difference is between acute and chronic pain; and how to get good information about pain relief and drugs.

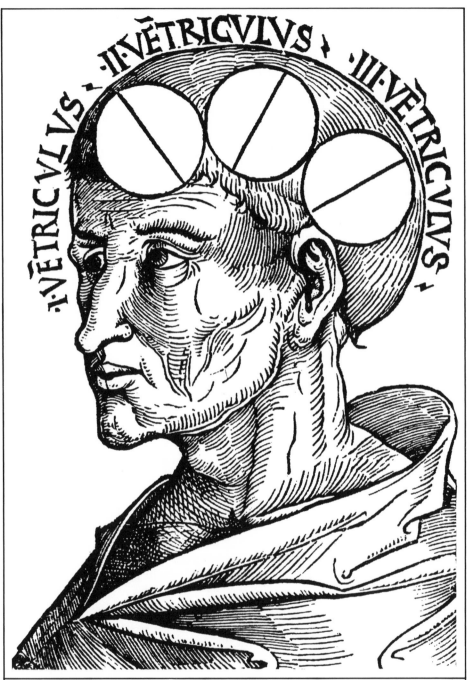

A 15th-century representation of the brain. One of the breakthroughs of modern neuroscience involves the knowledge that pain is processed and "felt" in the brain's thalamus and cerebral cortex.

CHAPTER 1

PAIN: IT'S MAINLY IN THE BRAIN

I have stood here before
inside the pouring rain,
with the world turning circles
running 'round my brain.
I guess I'm always hoping
that you'll end this reign,
but it's my destiny
to be the King of Pain.

—"King of Pain"
Words and music by Sting (Gordon Sumner)

Rock fans probably know that Sting's song poetically describes the universal awareness of pain — both physical and mental — among all living things. They may not appreciate that his lyrics also suggest connections between pain and the brain — connections that have come to be recognized in a stunning body of scientific knowledge.

For while pain may be sparked by a variety of things in a variety of places in and on the body, the triggers always send signals through ultra-thin nerve endings to the brain. And it is in the brain — specifically in the thalamus and the cerebral cortex—that pain is "felt." It is there that it "reigns."

It has taken many years but scientists at last know why it hurts when we smash a finger with a hammer or have a toothache. They have begun to make sense of the complicated sensations, processed in the brain, that we label simply "pain."

A look back at what people used to be told about why they felt pain helps us appreciate just how far science has advanced. Before neuroscientists developed their evidence for the brain-pain connection, a number of other theories of pain's origins were popular.

Prominent among these was the idea that noxious substances in the body, or evil "humors," poisoned the blood and caused disease and pain. American Plains Indian tribes were among many that blamed pain on demons who entered the body part that hurt. Practitioners of voodoo believe they can inflict pain at a distance. Ancient Chinese traditional medicine holds that disease and pain may arise when the two basic life principles, yin (negative, dark, feminine) and yang (positive, light, masculine), are out of balance.

The most persistent theories, however, attributed pain and disease to defects of moral or spiritual character. (It is no accident that the English word "pain" has the same root as the Latin and Greek words for "penalty.")

The notion that people in pain deserve their pain, that their pain is punishment by angry gods for sin and wrongdoing, is still part of many traditional and religious beliefs. Offshoots of these theories involve "mind over matter" philosophies that prescribe peace of mind through spiritual understanding to overcome pain. Fakirs (Muslim religious beggars) who walk on nails or hot coals and religious groups that forbid the use of medication are subscribers to these theories.

Centuries ago, blaming the victims for their suffering was certainly a convenience for healers who could not make the pain go away. On the other hand, such theories of the origins of pain would not have survived had there not been some basis for them.

Managing Stress and Anxiety

The basis for the "victims deserve their pain" theory concerns the body's reaction to stress and anxiety. The release of hormones and other biochemicals triggered by stress can in fact increase the intensity, duration, and perception of pain. Thus, those who strongly believe that the source of pain is not physical — shamans (priests of shamanism, a religion that holds that the world is pervaded by good and evil spirits that can be called forth by inspired individuals acting as mediums), priests, spiritualists, faith healers, for example — can often, in fact, relieve pain. They use chants, rituals, prayer, and other strategies designed to appease the gods, help sinners atone—and otherwise reduce fear and stress.

This kind of relief operates on the same principle most of us have observed when a small child is hurt and comes crying for relief. When we comfort or distract him (with a cookie, a toy, a cartoon), the child relaxes and seems far better able to tolerate pain or medical treatment. Psychologists and neuroscientists are in fact using their growing knowledge of the effects of stress on body chemistry to develop whole new approaches to treating pain and disease (see Chapter 8).

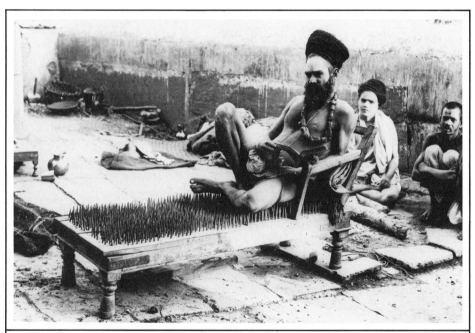

A Hindu fakir (holy beggar) from eastern India sits on a couch of nails. According to his religion, overcoming pain by mental discipline is a sign of spiritual growth and understanding.

By the 17th century Western scientists and philosophers began to look for pain's origins among the findings of anatomists (those who study the parts of the body) and physiologists (those who study bodily processes) to investigate pain's origins. These individuals were learning a great deal about tissues, organs, nerves, and the brain. They developed increasingly accurate pictures of the brain and spinal cord and their role in governing the body's movement and other activities.

In 1644 the French philosopher and mathematician René Descartes suggested that when a person's foot was burned the burning sensation yanked nerves attached to the brain and signaled it to react to the pain and danger of the fire.

For three centuries scientists built on Descartes's insights, and in the 20th century we know a great deal about the way burns and other painful stimuli send signals to the brain, how the brain recognizes those signals, what the brain does next, and what happens biochemically and physiologically throughout the entire complicated process.

A Complex Chain of Events

Researchers have discovered that pain is transmitted by a chain of electrical, chemical, and biological events in the body and the brain. Whenever damage occurs in the body, nerves in the affected area relay a stream of electrical impulses via chemical transmitters, called *neurotransmitters*, through the spinal cord to the thalamus, the part of the brain that receives such signals. The brain immediately communicates the pain and the danger, triggering the victim's automatic move to pull back from the source of the pain.

Pain experts have mapped the body's network of pain nerves, distinguishing it from the network that reacts merely to touch or pressure. They have identified the neurotransmitters in the brain, spinal cord, and elsewhere that control traffic along the network of pain nerves. In the last few years, scientists have also identified specific biochemicals — enzymes, hormones, and proteins — that are responsible for particular stops along the way to pain.

British scientist John Hughes, Hans Kosterlitz of the University of Aberdeen in Scotland, and Solomon Snyder of Johns Hopkins University unified many ideas about the brain, pain, and pain relief with their discovery that the brain has special recognition devices called receptors that evolved to handle the body's own opiatelike painkilling chemicals called enkephalins and endorphins. These findings led to an explosion of new studies and knowledge.

Components of Pain

Overall, pain has four separate parts.

The first is sometimes called *nociception*, the nervous system's first detection of damage to some tissue.

Nociceptors are the primary pain-sense receivers, specialized thin pain nerve endings attached to some of the 15 billion nerve cells, or neurons, in the human body. In one form or another, they are found in the skin, muscle, and internal organs of the body. Some are exquisitely sensitive to pressure, others to sharp blows or heat. Others respond to a tiny pinprick while ignoring the burn of a flame. In short, nociceptors located throughout the body are the first to transmit information about pain — its intensity and location — to the brain. They can sort out the different sensations produced by a prick, a sharp stab, and a burn.

When a person has a wisdom tooth pulled, develops a headache, or succumbs to a half nelson in a wrestling match, nociceptors are activated to send a stream of electrical and chemical signals into the central nervous system even before the person manages to yell "Ouch!" (The central nervous system is composed of the brain and spinal cord. Nerves that branch out to other parts of the body are known as the peripheral nervous system.)

Whether the first stimulus comes from outside or inside, the firing of sensory pain nerves that carry information from outside the central nervous system to the spinal cord and into the brain always starts with irritation and damage to a nerve ending.

Just how internal organs, deep inside the body and away from nerve pain receptors, signal "pain" to the brain is not fully understood, but scientists believe that cells in these organs "refer" their stimuli to nerve cells that relay pain impulses.

In any case, soon after the first signals are fired, tissue damage occurs and sensory pain fibers start firing at a rapid

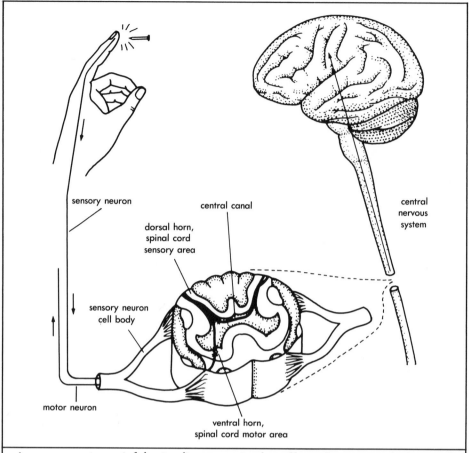

In response to painful stimuli, nerves in the affected area send electrical impulses to the brain via neurotransmitters along the spinal cord. The brain immediately communicates pain to the affected body part and triggers a move to withdraw from the source of pain.

rate. The second step in the pain process — perception of the pain itself — is launched when certain chemicals are released at the site of the injury and elsewhere. These chemicals cause the pain fibers to fire and also produce the heat, redness, swelling, and throbbing that we associate with many injuries.

Three of these chemicals are prostaglandins, substance P, and bradykinin. Prostaglandins are a group of substances linked to cramping and muscle pain.

Substance P is a large protein molecule that causes long spinal cord nerves in a multilayered structure called the dorsal horn to fire. Recent studies by Allan Basbaum and Jon Levine at the University of California in San Francisco show

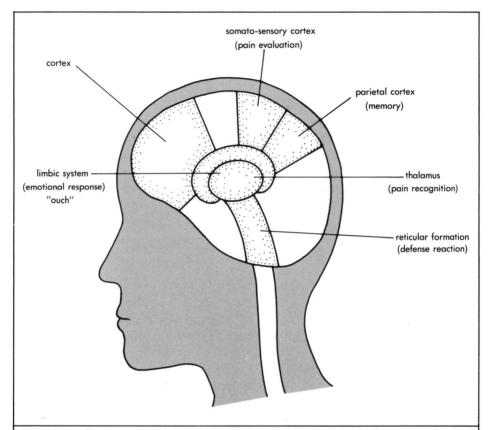

Pain signals are carried by nerve fibers along the spinal cord to two key "switching stations" in the brain. The first is the reticular formation at the lower end of the brain stem; the second is the thalamus. Ultimately, pain information reaches the cerebral cortex.

that substance P is released both inside the spinal cord and at the site of tissue injury, where it can keep reactivating pain nerves. Basbaum and Levine believe that the pain of arthritis, a chronic inflammation of the joints, occurs when pain nerves restimulate themselves this way.

Bradykinin, a product of the chemical reaction that occurs when blood vessels in damaged tissue break, is the most potent pain-producing substance known. Studies by Snyder and others at the Johns Hopkins University School of Medicine show that minute amounts of this peptide produce agonizing pain. They also discovered evidence that pain neurons in skin have specialized receptors for bradykinin, (just as the brain has special neuron receptors for opiate painkillers) proving bradykinin's role in initiating pain and possibly in enhancing the sensitivity of nociceptors. Bradykinin appears to be the real culprit in certain kinds of peripheral pain — sunburn, headaches, and arthritis — that do not respond to morphine and other narcotics.

Bradykinin also stimulates the release of prostaglandins, which in this case behave like secondary messengers that transmit electrical impulses through pain nerve cells to the brain. Aspirin, incidentally, works by blocking chemicals that form prostaglandins; it blocks the messenger rather than the real source, bradykinin.

Pathways of Pain

After firing, pain signals are carried by nerve fibers along the spinal cord to two key "switching" stations in the brain. The first is at the very top of the spinal cord or lower end of the brain stem; it is called the reticular formation. The second is the thalamus, a walnut-sized organ deep inside the base of the brain that functions like a relay station.

From here, pain information is further processed and signals are relayed to the highest level of the brain, the cerebral cortex, where pain is "felt" and its emotional consequences experienced.

Pain signals continue to travel to areas around the thalamus. Here, the brain has a large supply of opiate receptors and a rich supply of cells that produce enkephalins. Along with nerve impulses that originate in the brain and travel down the spinal cord, this system plays a key role in pain control, sending "Stop, pain!" signals down the track.

As mentioned earlier, traffic up and down the central nervous system is regulated by the release of chemicals called neurotransmitters, which cause nerve impulses to jump from the ending, or axon, of one nerve cell across a tiny gap, or synapse, to the dendrite of another nerve cell.

Neurotransmitters produce many effects. They can cause neurons to speed up or slow down the rate at which they fire signals across synapses, they can turn signals on and off, and they can operate alone or together to produce a variety of messages at the same time. In the late 1970s studies by a

Swedish scientist, Tomas Hokfelt, found that each neuron can release more than one transmitter, perhaps two or three. When released together, these "co-transmitters" work together to convey new and subtler information than would be transmitted by either a single chemical or the firing of single chemicals one at a time.

Four important neurotransmitters are acetylcholine, dopamine, norepinephrine, and epinephrine. These last two are also hormones and are released from the adrenal glands near the kidneys as well as in the brain. In their hormonal form they increase the heart rate, blood pressure, and the flow of sugar into the blood — all part of the "fight or flight" response to danger and injury that occurs in all animals and humans.

Our biological response to pain is clearly and closely linked to our response to danger. In Snyder's laboratory at Johns Hopkins, scientists have found special enzymes, or chemical catalysts, that play a role in the body's internal strategies against pain.

The third of pain's four components is what we often call suffering — our reaction to pain. As the thalamus interprets the chemically regulated electrical impulses as pain, these messages pass to other, higher levels of the brain. These include the limbic system, a strip of brain tissue around the thalamus that is responsible for emotional responses. At this point the person usually reacts with a yell, tears, fear, anxiety, or depression.

The impulses also go to various parts of the cortex, the outermost layers of the brain responsible for memory, pain assessment, and physical movement. Finally, they reach the pituitary gland and the hypothalamus, parts of the brain that also release endorphins and enkephalins, respectively, to ease pain from any source.

The fourth component of pain is what John D. Loeser of the University of Washington in Seattle calls "pain behavior." This, he says, is "anything a person says or does or does not do that would lead one to infer that a [painful] stimulus has occurred." Like all kinds of behavior, pain behaviors are influenced by past experience and outside factors that are not directly related to the origin of the pain. This component is often used to help explain why some people and even whole cultures and societies seem better able to tolerate pain than others.

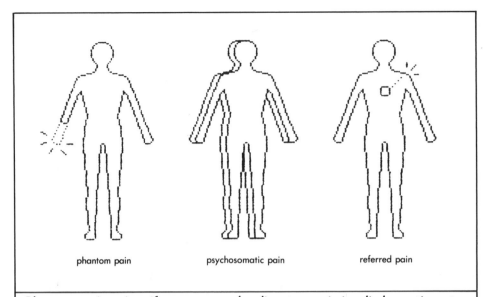

| phantom pain | psychosomatic pain | referred pain |

Phantom pain arises if nerves once leading to a missing limb continue to send messages to the brain. Psychosomatic pain feels like physical pain but is produced by anxiety and stress. Referred pain is sensed in an area other than one where actual damage has occurred.

Types of Pain

Many studies concerning the origins of pain have involved animals, which have simpler and more easily understood neurological systems than those of humans. This research has been able to classify various kinds of pain and distinguish levels of pain intensity.

Pain can be acute (usually short-lived and with a quickly identifiable trigger), chronic (the kind that lasts a long time and recurs), or psychosomatic (arising from mental or emotional factors).

Phantom pain seems to occur in an amputated limb because nerves that once served the missing part continue to send messages to the brain.

Referred pain occurs when the pain pathways literally get signals crossed. Pain is then felt at an area distant from the body part that has in fact been damaged. A common example is angina, in which victims of injury to the heart muscle often feel pain in the arm and neck.

What is the "worst" pain? Physicians, patients, and pain specialists generally agree that bone and deep-organ cancer pain, migraine, childbirth, phantom limb pain, and facial nerve conditions such as tic douloureux (literally: "painful tic," an intensely painful inflammation of certain facial nerves) are all candidates. But for someone in pain, the answer is clearly, "Mine."

There is still much to be learned about pain and pain transmission. Where, for example, does the first stimulus for a headache occur? We do not understand — biologically — why and how placebos (substances that look like drugs but contain no medication; they are administered for their psychological effects) work with some people and not others or exactly how stress and anxiety can trigger psychosomatic pains that are physically and chemically the same as those caused by physical injury. We also do not understand at precisely what stage an unborn baby develops the ability to perceive pain and what influences pain perception in infancy and childhood. Researchers continue their studies, however, and are certain to add to what is already a vast knowledge of the origins and mechanics of pain.

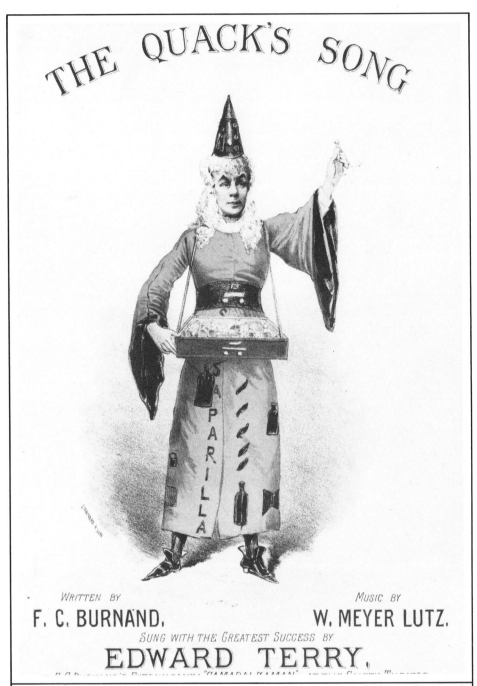

THE QUACK'S SONG

WRITTEN BY
F. C. BURNAND,

MUSIC BY
W. MEYER LUTZ.

SUNG WITH THE GREATEST SUCCESS BY
EDWARD TERRY,

A song from a bygone era deals with the theme of quackery. A boon of modern pharmacology is that there are now effective pain relievers; the quack's useless nostrums are largely a thing of the past.

CHAPTER 2

PAINKILLERS THEN AND NOW

The variety of ways in which pain tortures people is rivaled only by the variety of ways in which people have tried to relieve it.

Folk Remedies

From candles and copper bracelets to voodoo dolls and rubs and roots, treatments for pain have run the gamut of imagination. Cherokee Indians attempted to suck pain out through wood pipes, and American doctors before the Civil War used metal sticks to "draw out" the pain. Talismans (objects believed to have magical or protective powers) made of everything from garlic to garter snakes are still popularly used in some parts of the world to keep painful afflictions away.

Not all these methods — old or new — are without value. Copper, which was long believed to be an old wives' remedy for joint pain, may in fact interfere with the complex transmission of pain-nerve impulses.

Many ancient therapies survive today because trial-and-error experimentation — often driven by desperation — worked to some degree.

Acupuncture, the technique of inserting needles into certain points in the skin, is a good example of such a therapy. There is some evidence that the mild irritation caused by the needles activates nociceptors and stimulates the release of

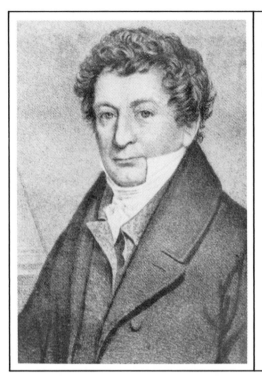

The German scientist Frederick Serteurner isolated morphine from the poppy plant in the early 19th century. This discovery quickly revolutionized the practice of medicine.

endorphins. Mild anesthetics such as camphor and peppermint are useful in soothing eczema (a red, itchy skin rash) and heating the chest to ease breathing. In ancient days, witch hazel and other oils were used to heal aches and treat cuts. They are still found in first-aid kits in many homes.

In 43 C.E. (C.E., or common era, is the same as A.D.), Scribonius Largus, a Roman physician, prescribed electric fish such as eels and torpedos for migraine and gout. This technique has a modern—and safer—equivalent in electrical stimulators that send a mild current through the skin to interrupt pain-nerve impulses.

Alcohol, mandrake root, opium, cannabis (marijuana), and coca have all been drunk, inhaled, chewed, smoked, or injected for centuries to numb or relieve pain. Heat, cold, and hypnosis, a trance-like state in which the subject is unusually receptive to suggestion, have all had their day and still have their uses. Massage in the form of osteopathy and chiropractics first became popular in the 1880s and brings temporary pain relief to millions with skeletal aches and pains.

Some methods are best forgotten, of course. Trephination — the practice of drilling a hole into the skull to let out painful fluids or humors — usually killed pain by killing the patient. Bloodletting with leeches and suction cups was often more painful than the source of the patient's own pain, and debilitating as well. Various scoundrels touting electromagnetic boxes, X rays, eyeball "vibrators" (for headaches), and water cures regularly duped a gullible public in the late 19th and early 20th centuries. Fortunately, such outrageous quackery is also by and large a thing of the past.

The use of drugs to stop pain traces its heritage to the craft of shamans, herbalists, and midwives. Until the 19th century, that heritage was about all science had to offer. Doctors in those days had little more to provide against severe pain than sympathy or the chemical equivalent of a knockout. The notion that substances could be made that would consistently and predictably relieve particular pains without further harming the patients or rendering them unconscious was still a dream.

The Birth of Modern Medicine

That dream began to be transformed to reality in 1806 when the German scientist Frederick Serteurner isolated the chemical morphine from the opium plant. Within 20 years of this achievement, morphine changed the practice of medicine. In fact, by the middle of the 19th century morphine was used throughout the United States and Europe to relieve virtually every type of pain.

In addition, by the 1840s scientists in Europe and the United States built on earlier experiments with gases by such men as Antoine-Laurent Lavoisier, a French chemist, and Joseph Priestley, a British clergyman, to develop anesthetics such as nitrous oxide (laughing gas) and ether. These gases, which control pain by rendering users unconscious or forgetful, were initially used almost exclusively for stage and party entertainments — anesthetized actors and participants behaved hilariously and without inhibition. In the years just before the American Civil War, however, several scientists realized that the sleep-inducing effects the gases had on those performing on stage might mean that these gases could also serve as an effective anesthetic.

Crawford Long, a country practitioner; William Morton, a Boston dentist; Horace Wells, for a brief time Morton's partner; and Charles Jackson, also a dentist; all played roles in the discovery of inhalation anesthesia.

In 1846 Morton effectively used ether as an anesthetic on a patient undergoing surgery for the removal of a tumor. His dramatic demonstration prompted its use by physicians and surgeons and stimulated the search for other means of painless surgery. Chloroform, another early inhalation anesthetic, was discovered in 1847. Healers began to experiment with ways of standardizing pain relief, making it safe and easy to use in the hospital, the backwoods, or on the battlefield.

Just as advances in anatomy, chemistry, and the scientific method helped usher in "general" or "put-you-to-sleep" anesthetics in the mid-19th century, they also led to interest in painkilling drugs besides morphine.

In 1857 cocaine, the active ingredient in coca, was isolated from the plant's leaf, the first step toward the scientifically based clinical application of the drug. First used as a topical anesthetic (local anesthetic applied directly to part

A 19th-century advertisement for a laughing gas (nitrous oxide) exhibition. The medical use of this drug as a general anesthetic came only after it had been widely used for novelty entertainments.

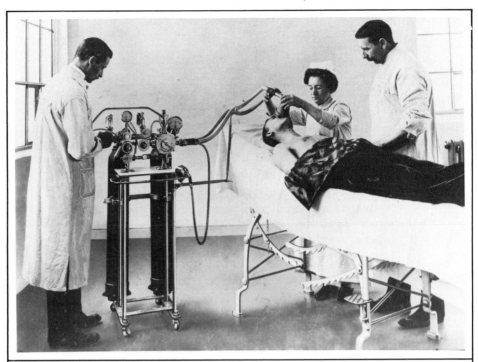

Inhalation anesthesia is administered to a surgical patient. By the 1840s, scientists were developing such anesthetics as nitrous oxide and morphine to relieve the pain of surgery.

of body being treated) for eye surgery by Carl Koller, a colleague of Sigmund Freud, and soon after for local "nerve block" by Johns Hopkins surgeon William Halsted, cocaine is regularly used today for throat, mouth, and nose surgery in major medical centers the world over. Able to block the transmission of nerve signals, cocaine is similar in this respect to alcohol and barbiturates.

The success of cocaine and increased attention to anesthesia and analgesia (loss of sensation of pain without loss of consciousness) predictably launched interest among slick entrepreneurs who took advantage of new manufacturing, packaging, and distribution schemes to mass market "patent" medicines. Particularly after the Civil War, these nostrums — including early versions of Coca-Cola — flourished. Most — such as Kick a poo Indian Sagwa and Dr. Pemberton's French Wine of Coca — contained a great deal of alcohol, opium, morphine, or codeine. When purveyors of these products boasted that they "cured all that ailed you" or were a "panacea" for pain, their users were hard put to find the lie through their drunken or drugged fog.

A major step toward safe analgesia came in 1830, when the active ingredient in willow bark — known for centuries to reduce fever and pain when steeped in tea — was isolated and synthesized in the chemical laboratory. Salicylic acid, in a form called acetylsalicylic acid, or aspirin, made Germany's Bayer Company world famous and wealthy.

By the turn of the century chemists working with synthetic (man-made) drugs were creating new analgesics with a variety of painkilling properties almost every year.

It may seem ironic that the flow of dubious or dangerous pain relievers and cure-alls into the marketplace reached flood-tide levels at the same time that the scientific foundations of drug development and use were emerging. In part, the problem was one of education. The public was still uncritical of drugs because they were unaware of or did not yet understand what physicians and others were beginning to discover.

The extent of widely accepted painkiller abuse probably reached an all-time high in the first decade of the 20th century. The first attempt to regulate drug use (1906 Wiley Pure Food and Drug Act) required only that drug labels state the amount of alcohol, morphine, opium, heroin, cocaine, chloroform, marijuana, and other substances in them.

"Soothing syrups" containing enough morphine to get a user jailed in the 1980s were fed daily to infants for the pain of colic, thereby addicting them. Laudanum (an opium preparation) and similar concoctions were so frequently prescribed to women for menstrual cramps and other gynecological problems that the addiction rate was four times higher among women than men despite the 400,000 Civil War soldiers estimated to have become addicted during treatment of their wounds.

In 1914 Congress passed the Harrison Act in an effort to regulate the rampant use of narcotics. This law required every doctor to have a license number to prescribe a narcotic and every pharmacist to obtain the number before filling the prescription. That system remains in place today.

By the early 20th century the stock of pain relievers used in and out of surgery included such anesthetics as cocaine, novocaine, stovaine, curare, halothane, Ethrane, and

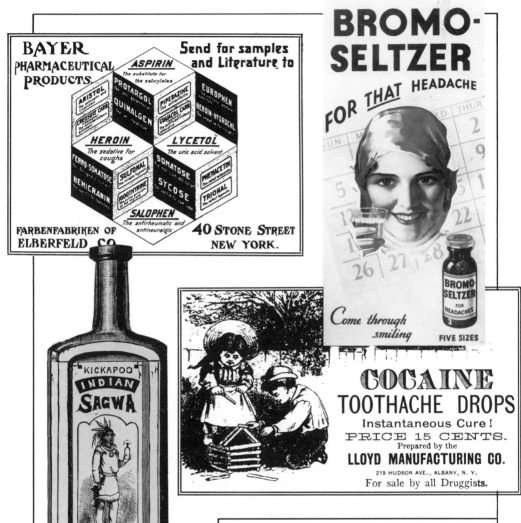

Four of the multitude of patent medicines readily available in the 19th and early 20th centuries. Some—aspirin products such as Bayer and Bromo-Seltzer —have become standard painkillers. Others, long since banned, contained heroin, cocaine, or morphine.

scopolamine. (Scopolamine mixed with morphine was a popular method of reducing pain in childbirth well into the 1970s; it put women in labor in a sort of "twilight" sleep, during which they experienced pain but could not remember it.)

New methods in the administration of anesthetics (caudal — injection into the extreme end of the spinal column — and spinal blocks, for instance) were also developed. In the 1980s, doctors have access to whole new classes of drugs, including steroids, nonsteroidal anti-inflammatory drugs, antiprostaglandins, antihistamines, narcotics, and drugs that block the release of bradykinins.

Not all pain relievers used in the 1980s are legal, and not all of their effects are understood or proven. Marijuana, for example, has mild analgesic effects in some people but not others. Barbiturates, like opiates, do not alter the perception of pain but do change a user's response to it. (Professional athletes are among the major abusers of barbiturates for this reason—to "play through their pain.")

Clearly, however, pain can be stopped with a variety of natural and synthetic drugs, taken either alone or in combination with others. In addition, there are some mood-altering drugs that help patients deal with pain by lowering their fears and raising their expectations that relief is in sight.

Limits of Regulation

A big factor in the widespread use of painkilling drugs today is the confidence people have in the products sold in the Western world.

Americans inject, swallow, inhale, or apply an astonishing array of pain relievers with a large degree of certainty that they will work as advertised. The Food and Drug Administration (FDA) and other government agencies regulate the claims manufacturers make, requiring warning labels on dosages and potential side effects. For the first time in history, patients and doctors alike have some measure of trust in the safety and value of the pain relievers they use.

To buy that trust and safety, however, Americans paid with some loss of marketplace and self-medicating freedom. With regulations came restriction and a growing social concern for the side effects of painkillers — euphoria, addiction, and withdrawal symptoms — that went beyond anything foretold on the warning labels on the pill bottle.

Although product regulation was directed at the issues of drug effectiveness and safety, it did not address the issue of how to deal with those individuals who used drugs primarily for their nonmedicinal side effects or became addicted or dependent upon them through a legitimate need for pain relief.

As a result, new ethical, social, moral, and legal issues joined the ancient drive for freedom from pain. Pain would no longer be an issue solely between the sufferer and those who sought to relieve suffering. Some societies, in fact, have outlawed potent pain relievers because of their undesirable side effects, while others have not. In the 1980s, for example, there is no legal use of heroin in the United States, whereas in England heroin is used for the pain of terminal cancer. Legalization of THC, the active ingredient in marijuana, used in cancer therapy against nausea and pain, was hard-won and is still hotly debated. Needless to say, it is still illegal to buy marijuana on the street or smoke it.

While these policies are viewed by some as unfair, history has taught some harsh lessons about safety and drugs. In 1806 the world hailed Serteurner's discovery of morphine, a potent painkiller reported to solve the "problem" of opium addiction. Morphine, of course, turned out to be as addictive as its predecessor, just as heroin, developed in the specific hope that it would have morphine's painkilling properties without its addicting properties, proved to be the principal substance of abuse for much of the 20th century.

Other, more recent painkillers have also proved addictive. Originally thought to be nonaddictive, the analgesic drug pentazocine (Talwin) was found to be addictive. Scientists hoped that fentanyl (Sublimaze), 100 times more potent than morphine, would be used so sparingly and with such control that addiction would be less likely. Studies show, however, that it is the principal narcotic of abuse among anesthesiologists and other physicians.

Even the body's own opiates, endorphins from the pituitary gland at the base of the brain and enkephalins from the brain itself, produce "tolerance" when production is overstimulated.

The age of scientific painkilling is upon us, but there is still no magic substance. All drugs, including those taken to relieve pain, have a downside. Narcotics, even in the service of healing, depress breathing and heart rate and sometimes strain the operation of other organs, such as the liver and kidneys. They alter brain function and biochemistry as well.

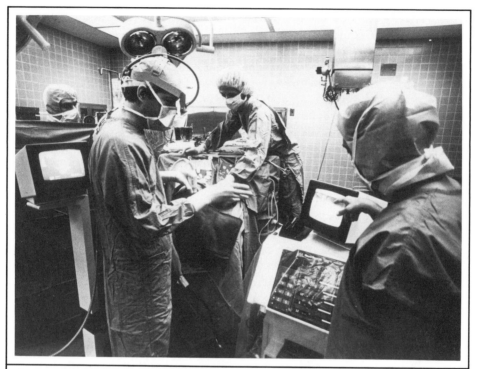

A neuroscientist uses ultrasound equipment to monitor the brain's activities in surgery. The development of sophisticated anesthetics for use during surgery is a success story of modern medicine.

Because no drug is without risk, relieving pain is always a balancing act. Caution is needed to prevent the risks from outweighing the benefits.

Furthermore, the dangers of painkilling substances are not limited to illegal and prescription drugs. Overdoses of "safe" over-the-counter analgesics, such as Tylenol, have occurred, causing permanent liver and kidney damage. Aspirin is associated with a fatal complication, Reye's syndrome, in children and teenagers recovering from flulike illness. Pain relievers can upset the digestive system, produce nausea, and jeopardize the development of the unborn.

Moreover, pain is a symptom, that is, an indication of a disease or injury. Pain relievers do not cure the underlying disease or heal an injury, but their use may mask pain symptoms that we need to experience in order to diagnose the underlying problem. Alcohol, barbiturates, narcotics, and anesthetics may so depress the central nervous system that unconsciousness and even death occur. Ergotamine, a potent weapon against migraine headache pain, can produce serious changes in brain chemistry and other adverse effects. Drugs such as tranquilizers and LSD that alter our perception of the world — including our pain — may permanently alter or damage brain tissue.

Nonetheless, no thoughtful person would argue that the potential abuse of pain relievers is reason to regret their discovery. Because pain continues to be a universal problem, the search for even more reliable, safe, and consistent pain relief continues.

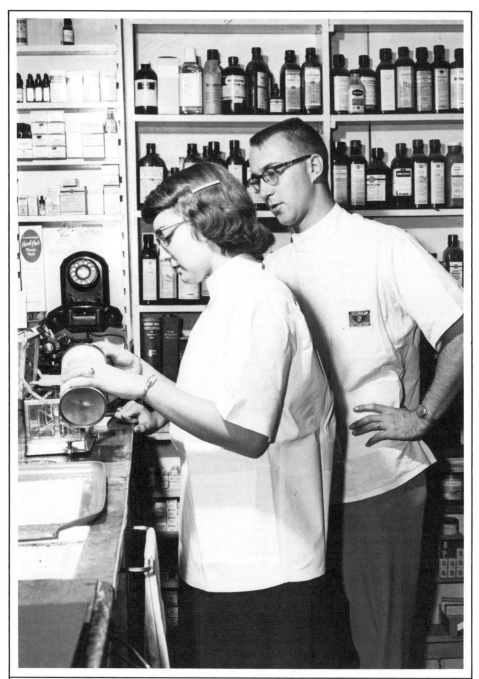

Modern pharmacies stock a wide variety of pain relievers. Although pharmacists fill prescriptions carefully, the consumer should always read and follow accompanying instructions for safety's sake.

CHAPTER 3

NONNARCOTIC ANALGESICS AND ANESTHETICS

Few would argue with the statement that to be safe, people seeking pain relief should use the least possible amount of the least potent substance to get the job done. Many people, however, believe that aspirin and other nonnarcotic analgesics are effective medicines for a cut finger or mild headache, but of little value against serious, long-term pain. So they escalate the war against pain with weapons that "overkill" the pain out of fear that anything less will fail to bring relief.

Fortunately, scientists — and increasingly nonscientists, too — are learning that many nonnarcotic analgesics are vastly underused and undervalued in the treatment of pain in adults and young people.

John Bonica, known to many as the father of modern pain treatment, has noted that with even a modest working knowledge of the duration and potency of analgesics, doctors can often successfully treat even severe pain effectively without resorting to narcotics and anesthetics.

To select the right pain medicine wisely, then, users need to understand how analgesics and anesthetics are classified.

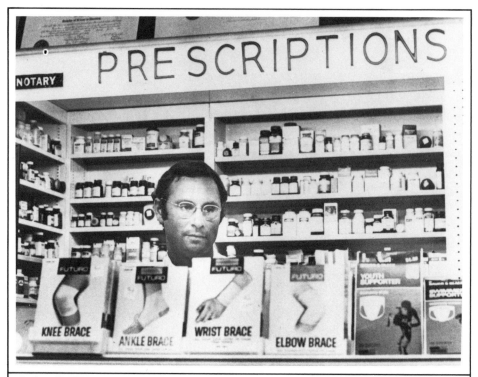

NOTARY

PRESCRIPTIONS

KNEE BRACE · ANKLE BRACE · WRIST BRACE · ELBOW BRACE

Only pharmacists may dispense prescription painkillers. However, many nonprescription drugs such as aspirin and ibuprofen are safe and effective analgesics if used properly.

Classifying Pain Relievers

One familiar method of classification is "prescription" versus "nonprescription." Prescription analgesics can be given only by doctors and are dispensed only by them or pharmacists. Many of these drugs are known as narcotics (from the word "narcosis," from the Greek for "to benumb") because they depress the central nervous system. They are also called opiates (see Chapter 4). Other, nonnarcotic analgesics are dispensed by prescription because they can cause side effects that need monitoring.

Nonprescription analgesics can be purchased over the counter in pharmacies, drugstores, and supermarkets. Studies ordered and evaluated by the FDA have declared them to be generally safe and effective when used as directed on the package.

Unfortunately, this classification is somewhat misleading. It wrongly suggests to many consumers that only "prescription" analgesics really work and that over-the-counter (OTC) medications are basically harmless, if not useless, against serious or nagging pain.

Neither situation is the case. OTC does not mean "harmless." All drugs must be taken with care, and, as mentioned, many OTC drugs have serious side effects in some people even with proper dosage. Many more are dangerous if abused, and abuse is easier when no prescriptions must be written.

A second way of classifying analgesics is by their site of action. Drugs that act on the peripheral nervous system — that is, outside the brain and spinal cord pathway — affect local receptors in skin and internal organs. Aspirin, which is both a pain reliever and reducer of inflammation and fever, is the most widely used and effective peripheral analgesic known, although it also has some central nervous system activity.

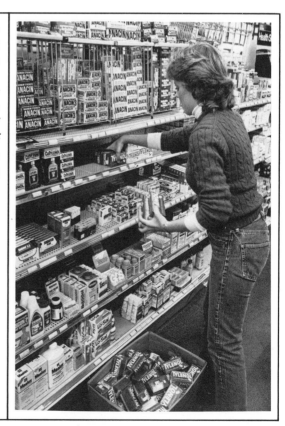

A wide range of over-the-counter medications is available to the consumer in supermarkets and drugstores. Unfortunately, many people assume that these preparations are "harmless," when in fact, a number of them can have serious side effects and are dangerous if abused.

Drugs that act mostly on the central nervous system (CNS) include morphine, heroin, meperidine (Demerol), and other narcotic analgesics. They work in areas that contain opiate receptors. Other CNS pain relievers include anesthetics such as nitrous oxide (laughing gas), antidepressants, tranquilizers, and anticonvulsants.

The third and best way for consumers to classify pain relievers is by their intended use: for mild, moderate, or severe pain.

In this system of classification, drugs used for mild to moderate pain include nonnarcotics and "weak" narcotics such as codeine. For severe pain, either combinations of these drugs or stronger narcotics may be used.

Anesthetics fit into this classification system as drugs that affect the central nervous system by preventing the perception of inflicted pain. These are properly used only to prevent pain during surgery. They include local or topical anesthetics, injected locally, that block local nerve impulses. These drugs are excellent against the pain of minor surgery such as tooth extraction, biopsies, or stitching up a deep cut. Specially trained anesthesiologists also can use them to treat certain conditions characterized by endlessly firing pain-nerve cells.

Other drugs whose uses are easier to sort out under this classification are sometimes known as "adjuvant" drugs. These enhance or add to the effectiveness of true analgesics and anesthetics but are not themselves true analgesics. Among them are tranquilizers, muscle relaxants, antidepressants, and mild hallucinogenics such as THC, the active ingredient in marijuana.

This kind of analgesic ladder — based on what analgesics are used for — not only takes into account the intensity of a person's pain, but also such factors as how the drugs are given (by mouth, injection), the effect of combinations of drugs to reduce addiction, dependence or side effects, and the use of combinations to both reduce required amounts and enhance pain relief.

With this system, doctors can account also for differences in such things as a patient's age in the selection of an analgesic. For example, with morphine, a potent narcotic, the effects last longer in older patients.

Another important benefit of this classification system is that it accurately illustrates the variety of choices available to relieve a particular kind of pain. There are far more than most people think.

It is reassuring to know that physicians have so many choices; if one does not work, others probably will. Pain relief is not a question of a knockout punch. The goal is to bring relief without doing harm. For this purpose, lightweights are often as effective as heavyweights, provided their handlers know a winning strategy.

The next chapter explains how the heavyweights work and how scientists are making them safer. The list below concentrates on the lower end of the analgesic ladder and on anesthetics — how they work and the kinds of pain each treats best.

Oral Analgesics for Mild to Moderate Pain

Aspirin (acetylsalicylic acid) in its many forms and combinations remains the most widely used, trusted, and predictable analgesic in the world. Thousands of tons are used annually. Aspirin products relieve nonmigraine headaches, joint pain, muscle cramps, and other mild to moderate pain as well as fever and inflammation. Aspirin is the drug of choice for tennis elbow, moderate menstrual cramps, toothaches, and surface cuts and burns.

Drug experts like to point out that if aspirin were to be discovered today, it would be hailed as a miracle drug because of its effectiveness against so many pains, fevers, cramps, and other maladies. It also would probably be available only by prescription and would be expensive as well.

Aspirin is made from salicin, the active ingredient in willow bark. The Bayer Company in Germany was the first — at the turn of this century — to find a synthetic derivative that did not overirritate the stomach; they called the substance aspirin.

In recent years scientists have learned that aspirin's main activity is its interference with the production of prostaglandins, the hormonelike substances produced by the body after tissue is injured. In 1982 Sune Bergstrom, Bengt Samuelsson, and John Vane won the Nobel Prize in Medicine for identifying the role of prostaglandins in pain and other bodily functions. Their discoveries, elaborated by others, show that aspirin stops pain by sabotaging the basic chemical building

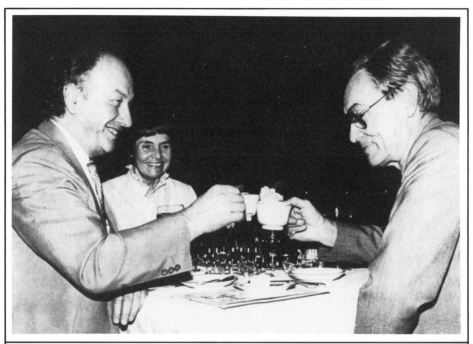

Sune K. Bergstrom, right, and John Vane toast each other after learning that they were part of a trio that won the 1982 Nobel Prize for Medicine. With Bengt Samuelsson, they successfully identified the role and functions of prostaglandins in the body.

blocks of prostaglandin in our cells. The production of prostaglandins is sparked by bradykinin, a potent pain nerve stimulant (see Chapter 1).

The pain-relieving powers of aspirin are often underrated. Studies show that a single dose (two tablets) can be equal to or better than such oral narcotics as propoxyphene (Darvon) and codeine. For the pain following childbirth or surgery, aspirin is as powerful as any painkiller that can be taken orally.

Some aspirin products contain more than the standard dose of aspirin (400 or more milligrams (mg) as opposed to 325 mg in the usual tablet), but studies show that increased doses are likely to increase the risk of side effects without adding to pain relief very significantly. In very large doses, aspirin can lead to serious complications, such as internal bleeding.

Acetaminophen works very much like aspirin to reduce pain and fever, but not inflammation. It has approximately the same pain-relieving properties as aspirin but in a substantial number of people is less effective.

Sold under such trade names as Datril, Tylenol, Liquiprin, and Tempra, acetaminophen is widely recommended for use by children under 16 years in place of aspirin for headache, fever, and simple muscle and joint pains. The reason is safety: as we have said, aspirin has been linked to an increased risk of Reye's syndrome, a sometimes fatal complication of viral illnesses such as chicken pox and flu. Although aspirin has not been clearly shown to be a cause of Reye's, its association with the syndrome has been enough to warrant warning labels on aspirin packages and recommendations by the American Academy of Pediatrics that children use acetaminophen during and after viral illness.

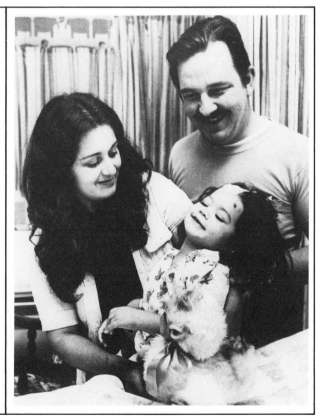

A victim of Reye's syndrome — a potentially fatal complication of the chicken pox or flu — shows signs of recovery in a California hospital. Studies have concluded that children who take aspirin during and after certain viral illnesses increase their risk of contracting Reye's syndrome.

Chemically classified as a nonsteroidal anti-inflammatory drug, ibuprofen is one of the newest of the nonnarcotic, nonprescription oral pain relievers on the market. It was first sold under the name Motrin as a prescription drug for joint inflammation and severe menstrual cramping. In the 1980s, under names such as Nuprin and Advil, it is also sold over the counter as 200- to 400-mg tablets and has a higher potential than aspirin for fast, long-acting pain relief for mild to moderate pain.

Because ibuprofen is not the same chemical formulation as aspirin, it is recommended especially for the very small percentage of people who are allergic to aspirin and those whose stomachs are irritated by aspirin and aspirin products.

Other nonsteroidal anti-inflammatory agents, such as Phenylbutazone (marketed under the trade name Butazolidin) and indomethacin, relieve inflammation of joints in arthritis and after accidental injury. In this way, they do relieve pain, but because these prescription drugs do not have a direct analgesic effect, and because they may cause blood and metabolic problems, they are not used very often for pain relief in the absence of serious inflammation.

Steroids such as *prednisone* and *cortisone* — both prescription drugs — also reduce pain caused by inflammation of damaged joints. Again, because they can have serious side effects (such as serious weight gain and kidney and liver damage) and mask tissue pain and damage without healing, their use is not recommended for routine aches and pains.

Cannabis, or marijuana, has a long reported history of mild analgesic effect and has long been used by various cultures as a muscle relaxer. It is not known, however, whether these effects are biological or psychological. Given the drug's illegal status and habit-forming properties, its use for pain-relieving purposes is unjustified, except under those rare conditions when its use is prescribed by a physician.

Anesthetics

There are two types of "general" anesthetics, or drugs that induce sleep, stupor, or extreme euphoria. Neither of these types directly stops pain; rather, both prevent the perception or experience of pain. The first are inhalation anesthetics, or gases, and include ether, nitrous oxide, and cyclopropane.

The form of ether used in anesthesia is ethyl oxide or diethyl ether. It is a thin, colorless, highly volatile, and highly flammable liquid. Widely used in general anesthesia (complete sedation), ether goes to work more slowly than most other general anesthetics. Nitrous oxide, also known as laughing gas for the effect it has on recipients, acts on central nervous system structures in a way similar to narcotics. Its pain-relieving properties are considerable, and it triggers a euphoric "high." Cyclopropane is another gaseous anesthetic agent. It is colorless and slightly heavier than air.

The second kind of general anesthetic is called intravenous because it is injected into a vein. The best known of these drugs is sodium pentathol.

Both inhalation and intravenous anesthetics cause a rapid loss of consciousness and pain sensation and, in smaller doses, a loss of inhibitions. Deep general anesthesia for surgical procedures brings on a complete loss of consciousness, spinal cord function, cell movement, and muscle tension. Anesthetics slow down breathing and heart rate, some brain activity, and metabolism.

Pain relief for minor surgical procedures is simpler and safer with topical or "local" anesthetics such as cocaine, procaine (Novocain), and lidocaine. When injected into exposed tissue, they block nerves and numb the area while also relaxing nearby muscles.

For some kinds of surgery, anesthesiologists use combinations of anesthetics and analgesics to help reduce the risk of loss of consciousness brought on by sleep-inducing gases. Diazepam (Valium) is used for this purpose in many young people for extracting wisdom teeth. Curare, a deadly poison used for centuries by South American Indians to kill enemies, is, in the skilled hands of a specialist, an important muscle relaxant.

Many reflexes aggravate pain by keeping the entire pain cycle heated up. By blocking certain nerve pathways in the autonomic nervous system responsible for such "automatic" reflexes as heart rate and sweating, anesthesiologists can slow these reflexes down.

Finally, local anesthetics are injected into the spinal fluid around the spinal cord and numb the pelvic region. Such "spinal" or "caudal" anesthesia procedures became common

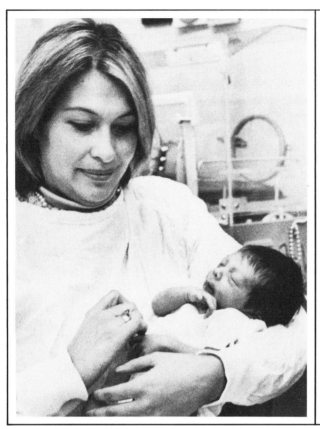

A mother enjoys her first contact with her healthy newborn. Epidural anesthetics, which relieve pain while still allowing a person to feel sensations, are a recent alternative to full spinal anesthetics during childbirth.

in the United States after World War II to lessen the pain of childbirth. More recently, doctors began to use epidural ("epi" means "around" — in this case around the spinal cord's fatty tissues) to deaden pain but permit women in labor to retain enough sensation to help "bear down" on pelvic muscles and keep the labor going.

Adjuvant Agents

Many drugs are used to enhance or extend the action of analgesics and anesthetics:

Diazepam (Valium) and minor tranquilizers often relieve the emotional stress and anxiety that aggravate pain. The minor tranquilizers may also enhance the action of morphine; the major tranquilizers, such as the phenothiazines, can be used with weak narcotics (Darvon, for example) to reduce the amount of narcotics needed to stop pain.

Tricyclic antidepressants, including amitriptyline, work especially well to increase the potency of weaker narcotics. Lithium, an element widely used to stop the violent mood swings of manic depressives, works in some patients to prevent cluster migraines, the most severe type of headaches.

Anticonvulsants used primarily to treat epilepsy also benefit many with pain caused by uncontrollable nerve abnormalities or damage. These conditions include tic douloureux.

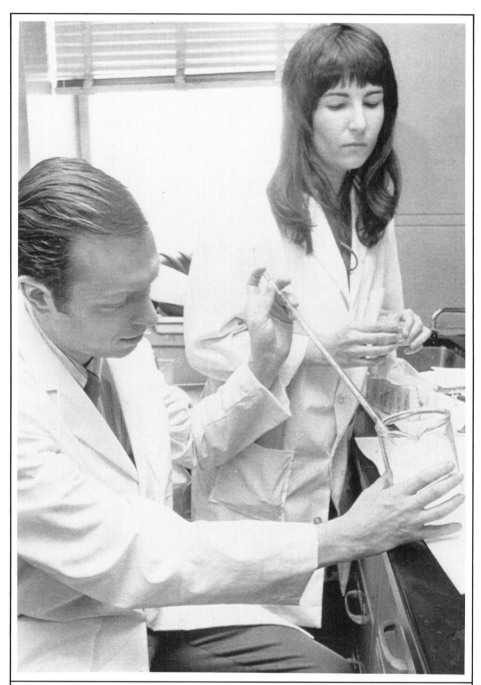

Drs. Solomon Snyder and Candace Pert in their laboratory at Johns Hopkins University. Their pioneering research unlocked many secrets about pain, how narcotics kill pain, and the mystery of addiction.

CHAPTER 4

NARCOTICS: THE LINK BETWEEN PLEASURE AND PAIN

Two bitter, white tablets bring relief to a teenager moaning with pain after a dental surgeon removes four wisdom teeth.

Physicians in a coronary care unit inject a liquid into an intravenous line; within moments, a young man immobilized with crushing chest pain feels better.

A high school soccer player writhes with pain and fear caused by an injury to his foot until an injection into his hip bathes him in peace and he sleeps.

To see firsthand the unmatched power of narcotics to relieve severe pain in a still-conscious person is, some say, to watch a miracle. The scene frequently inspires as much awe in the observer as relief in the patient. "Whenever I can stop terrible pain with these drugs," says one young doctor, "I feel my own tension vanish and sometimes I am so grateful, I am choked with tears."

This young doctor's visceral response occurs not because he gives his patients pleasure, but because he takes away their pain. The goal of the medical use of narcotics against pain is not euphoria, but analgesia — not the presence of joy, but the absence of agony.

Yet the two situations — absence of pain and presence of pleasure — are closely linked, not only in our minds and senses, but also in our biology, and narcotic analgesics have played a critical role in displaying the nature of those links in human beings.

In order to understand that role — and its implications for better, safer pain relief — it is necessary to know something about narcotics, where they come from, how they work, and why they are dangerously addictive.

The Origins of Narcotics

Thousands of years ago, healers first extracted milky fluid from the unripened seeds of the poppy (*Papaver somniferum*), a red-flowered plant native to Asia Minor that is the source of all natural narcotics. The fluid, called opium, from the Greek word for "juice," was used to relieve headaches, colic, gallstones, and the pain associated with wounds and surgery.

The use of opium in medicine was preserved by Islamic populations after the fall of the Roman Empire and was introduced by the Arabs to Persia, China, and India. By the 16th century it was widely known in Europe.

Opium contains at least 20 compounds, called alkaloids. Of these, a handful are pharmacologically active: morphine, codeine, and papaverine are the best known. (Confusion sometimes occurs about the inclusion of cocaine — chemically a stimulant — in lists of narcotics. The confusion occurs because in the Controlled Substances Act, cocaine is designated as a narcotic for purposes of scheduling — classifying drugs according to a system designed by the FDA — and law enforcement, as discussed in Chapter 7. Although cocaine, other stimulants, depressants, hallucinogens, and marijuana are habit forming and may result in physical dependence, they are not narcotics.)

Several years after Serteurner first isolated morphine, codeine was discovered. This narcotic is obtained from morphine, but is only one-sixth as potent.

Heroin — chemically known as diacetylmorphine because two acetyl groups were added to morphine to create it — was developed by the Bayer aspirin chemists in 1898. It is as much as 10 times more potent than morphine. Because it enters the brain more rapidly than morphine, giving the user a "rush" or "high," heroin has been the most sought-after narcotic among abusers.

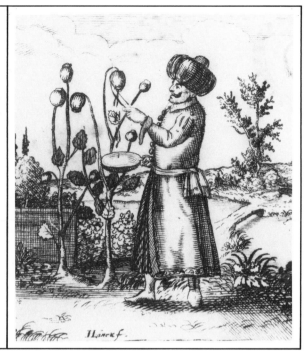

A 17th-century illustration shows a man slashing an opium bud. Although the modern narcotics derived from this plant are highly effective painkillers, they have also proven to be dangerously addictive.

Curiously, heroin's addictive properties went unrecognized for almost a quarter of a century after its development. One reason, according to drug experts and historians, may be that heroin was first used in cough syrups. Narcotics are powerful cough suppressants because they slow down many reflexes, including the one for coughing. However, it was difficult to get sufficient concentrations into the blood or brain via cough syrup to create a rapid rush or addiction. Moreover, the early uses of heroin were so strictly confined to medical treatment that users never *expected* a psychoactive effect.

Since people did not *expect* to get "high" on heroin, the drug was not really abused for many years, demonstrating once again the influence of social context and mental attitude on drug abuse. For example, studies show that dying cancer patients in severe pain use far fewer narcotics if they are permitted to take them whenever they feel the need than patients who must depend on someone else to administer the drugs. It was not long, however, before heroin was wedded to the hypodermic syringe (developed just before the Civil War), just as morphine had been earlier, and began to be abused.

Effects of Narcotics

The effects of narcotic analgesics are well known. With the exception of papaverine, which is used mainly as an anti-spasmodic (controlling spasms), all narcotics are central nervous system depressants, affecting body and mind.

Narcotics depress breathing, and cause nausea, drowsiness, loss of appetite, apathy, and a slowdown of all biological functions. They are also known, of course, for their ability to induce euphoria, tolerance, and the typical kind of addiction that results in watery eyes, irritability, tremors, panic, cramps, chills, and nausea when the drug is withdrawn. Narcotics can also damage the fetus of an addicted mother.

In overdoses, narcotics bring on shallow breathing, clammy skin, convulsions, shock, coma, and, possibly, death.

Because narcotics — whether they are natural (derived from opium) or synthetic — all result in similar effects and side effects, they are often referred to as "opiates."

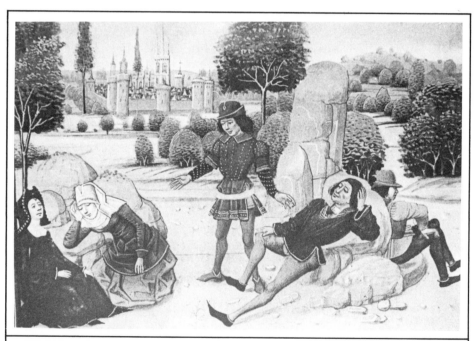

Morpheus, the Greek god of dreams, displays his powers in this medieval miniature. The drug morphine, which causes drowsiness when ingested, derives its name from this Greek deity.

The synthetic and semisynthetic narcotic analgesics, manufactured by manipulating the molecules found in the natural products, include hydromorphone (Dilaudid); meperidine (Demerol, Mepergan, Lomotil); methadone and its first cousins, including Darvon; pentazocine (Talwin); fentanyl (Sublimaze); and synthetic codeines (Percodan). These drugs are called opioids to recognize their man-made status, just as science fiction buffs call man-made people androids.

With the exception of heroin, all these drugs are used for medical purposes in the United States. Heroin, legal in Great Britain for medical use, is under investigation here for that purpose. Although narcotics have various routes of administration (codeine is usually taken orally and morphine by injection) and various rates of physical and psychological dependence, all these drugs are potentially addictive.

Anyone who would use a narcotic should be familiar with what normally happens in the body and brain after the drug is taken. In general, if it is injected into a muscle, the pain-relieving properties of an opiate start working about a half hour after it has been administered. Its effects peak within 90 minutes of a single safe dose. When a narcotic is injected into a vein, the effect may occur in seconds and peak a few minutes later.

By way of the bloodstream, the drug reaches such organs as the lungs and liver. Only a small amount travels to the brain, but it is enough to produce profound effects on our most protected organ.

After decades of studies, doctors have found that the optimal — or best and safest — dose of a narcotic for severe pain relief is generally 15 mg for a 150-pound man. All narcotics have profound sedative effects; all dilate blood vessels. All act similarly to morphine and differ among themselves mainly in the degree of their actions. As mentioned earlier, opiates depress the cerebral cortex, causing sleep, general depression, reduction in perception of pain, euphoria, reduced inhibitions, and reduced fear as they slow down the activity of the hypothalamus and brain stem.

Ironically, narcotics also temporarily stimulate the spinal cord, leading to nausea, vomiting, constipation, itching, yawning, and sweating. Users can also expect drowsiness, mental and physical impairment (it is extremely dangerous to drive under the influence of an opiate), and poor concentration.

Another dangerous effect of narcotics is the rapid development of "cross-tolerance." If a person becomes tolerant to morphine, that person is likely to become tolerant even faster to meperidine or fentanyl.

The most powerful narcotics — heroin, morphine, fentanyl, meperidine — are most useful in heart attacks (they treat pain, but also tranquilize and reduce the heart's oxygen-producing work load); just before or during surgical anesthesia, to enhance sedation and reduce fear; after surgery, to reduce pain and anxiety; and for the deep, dull pain of cancer.

Observations, Questions, and Hunches

Although opiates have been with us since ancient times, the *real* story of narcotics — *why* they work the way they do — unfolded only in the 1970s and 1980s. Moreover, that knowledge has uncovered nature's internal pain-relief schemes and opened the door to a new era in safer design of potent analgesics that kill pain without side effects or addiction.

The story begins, as do all advances in science, with observations, questions, and hunches.

Observation: A Canadian woman with a perfectly normal nervous system and brain (later confirmed on autopsy) feels absolutely no pain even when needles are inserted into her body, electric shocks are applied, and sticks are thrust up her nose. How is this possible?

Observation: Runners and other athletes exhibit every sign of intense pain as they push their bodies beyond the breaking point but report that either they do not notice the pain or finally "hit the wall" and break through to an intense sensation of pleasure and well-being. What accounts for this pleasure from pain?

Observation: The intense pleasure narcotic addiction brings to users is followed relatively rapidly by the intense pain of withdrawal. What goes on in the body to produce the flip-flop? Why would nature have evolved a brain that could be influenced so mightily by such natural products as the juice of a poppy?

Observation: Studies of the brain show that certain tissues in the brain absorb narcotics more quickly and more thoroughly than do other tissues in the brain. Why?

Observation: The ancient art of acupuncture — insertion

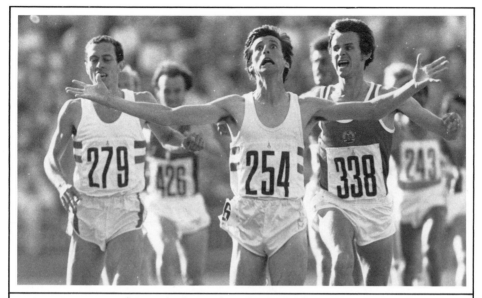

Runners report that a feeling of euphoria makes them oblivious to the pain induced by their exertions. Scientists speculate that a release of endorphins may be responsible for this "runner's high."

of needles into the skin at various places — is a potent analgesic and anesthetic for large numbers of Chinese and other individuals. What is going on?

Observation: As humans evolved, their ability to withstand great physical discomfort — from the elements, from injuries — played a great role in survival. In many societies and cultures, individuals seek out pain — in hunts, contests, and so on — in anticipation of the pleasure that apparently follows cessation of the pain. If the pleasurable consequences were not great, why would anyone ever engage in such behavior?

Observation: Some animals, including humans, even find pleasure in pain. These individuals are sometimes called masochists, and their behavior is condemned. But, is it possibly advantageous to the survival of our species that nature lets humans experience pain as sometimes rewarding?

Hunch: Humans have probably evolved one or more internal means of producing physical pleasure in response to painful stimuli.

Hunch: At least one of those mechanisms must involve the release of chemical messengers that very rapidly bathe the senses in pleasure or shut off painful stimuli. The ebb and flow of narcotic euphoria and withdrawal symptoms strongly suggest a subtle chemical/molecular basis for addiction rather than a gross mechanical one.

Hunch: It is likely that there are molecules within brain cells that attract or have an affinity for opiates. This idea is based on the fact that other brain chemicals fit like tiny "keys" into such "receptors," or "locks."

Many scientists were familiar with these observations, asked these questions, and had these hunches. In an attempt to find the brain's opiate receptors, for example, they ground brain tissue and mixed it with opiates that were "tagged" with radioactive tracers (so they could be located and counted with equipment similar to a Geiger counter).

The results of these tests, conducted as early as the 1950s, failed to show the presence of specific opiate receptors in the brain. The problem was that the number of receptors was so tiny — we know now they account for less than a millionth of the brain's weight — and the measuring devices were not sensitive enough.

The breakthrough came in the mid-1970s through the research of Doctors Solomon Snyder and Candace Pert of Johns Hopkins University School of Medicine. At the time, Snyder and Pert were looking for new ways to explore the effect of narcotics on the brain.

They reasoned that although opiates might bind to receptors, they might also bind with other tissues; the number of the "nonspecific" binding sites was thus likely to be greater than the number of specific receptor sites they were looking for.

Snyder and Pert found out how to separate the two by taking advantage of the fact that opiate receptors can detect and bind very low concentrations of opiates, and only in the vicinity of the receptors. They played to the *scarcity* of the receptors instead of fighting it.

The next step was logical and brilliant in its simplicity. Instead of using radioactive pure opiates, they used radioactive preparations of an opiate antagonist. In scientific terms, an agonist is an active substance, in this case the opiate. An antagonist is a substance that fights or neutralizes an agonist.

Emergency room doctors had known for years the value of naloxone, an opiate antagonist. When heroin addicts overdose, naloxone, if injected quickly enough, counteracts the effect of the opiate and prevents the lethal depression of breathing. The antagonist worked in the brain somehow to counteract the effect of the heroin.

Snyder and Pert theorized that if the antagonist did indeed work to help addicts by taking up the spaces in the receptors that are normally filled with the opiate, they could just as easily trace the long-sought opiate receptors through opiate antagonists as through the opiates themselves.

Using naloxone, they were able to add very tiny — but very detectable — amounts of the radioactive tags to ground-up brain tissue. The Hopkins team then removed any evidence of naloxone that was not bound tightly to other molecules. The molecules to which the naloxone bound were, in fact, the opiate receptors.

Then, they showed that the binding sites accounted for the effect of opiates by measuring the ability of nonradioactive opiates to compete with naloxone for the binding sites — a kind of molecular horse race. To their delight, they discovered a direct correlation between the amount of an opiate taken and the number of receptors in the brain to which that drug bound and to the amount of a drug doctors knew would relieve pain.

Snyder and Pert's feat would have been, in itself, a satisfying scientific and technical advance, but that was not the reason they won their Lasker Award and will, many believe, ultimately win a Nobel Prize for their work. Their achievement suggested an incredible new set of questions about brain chemistry and pain relief that could change forever the way pain is understood and treated.

For example, why would the brain have opiate receptors only to accommodate a few substances that had been known for less than a few thousand years? In the evolutionary history of humankind, what did those receptors evolve to do?

For Snyder and Pert, the answer seemed clear: the brain must have some of its *own* opiates, natural painkilling chemicals that substances such as morphine and heroin just happen to mimic.

Other observations and hunches would come together if this were so. For example, the survival advantages of such a chemical for prehistoric humans would be tremendous if they could numb their own pain when injured or exposed to harsh environments.

With this simple and highly accurate technique for identifying opiate receptors, Snyder and his team at Hopkins
quickly began to ask and answer many questions and make
many discoveries. Most of all they learned a great deal about
pain, how narcotics kill pain, and addiction.

They learned, for example, how agonists differed from
antagonists. (They broke down differently in the presence of
sodium.)

They pinpointed areas of the brain and spinal cord where
opiate receptors were located and showed there were dis-
tinct patterns that corresponded with what brain anatomists
had long identified as areas known to be involved in pro-
cessing pain signals.

They learned that at the spinal cord level, opiates relieve
pain by raising a person's tolerance to pain, but in the brain,
they work by dulling the brain's ability to read pain signals.
"Patients who have been treated with morphine," Snyder
notes, "because of severe postoperative discomfort or extreme pain from cancer frequently tell their doctors, 'It's a
funny thing. The pain is still there, but it doesn't bother me.' "

Snyder and Pert knew that another part of the brain, the
thalamus, conveys nerve signals linked to deep, burning, aching pain, the kind best relieved by narcotics. They were not
surprised to find intense concentrations of opiate receptors
there.

These scientists were able to explain the long-known
fact that there are two types of pain, fast and slow, signaled
by different kinds of nerve fibers. Opiates affect only slow
pain, and the researchers were able to show that this was
related to the locations of opiate receptors.

The Brain's Own Opiates

Undoubtedly, however, Snyder and Pert's biggest challenge
was to find, identify, and isolate the brain's own opiates, those
chemicals they *knew* must be there. The findings on opiate
receptors had made the search possible. Knowing where
these chemicals were likely to be, and in what concentrations,
gave the research team a shot at finding them.

In 1975, in Scotland, John Hughes and Hans Kosterlitz,
who were also attempting to find the opiate receptors, took
advantage of the fact that opiates influence intestinal con-

tractions. (Because of this property, narcotics are used to control diarrhea, among other medical problems.) If the brain indeed had an opiatelike chemical, or neurotransmitter, Hughes and Kosterlitz reasoned, it should then work on the intestine in the same way that opiates do. They were able to extract substances from pig brains that influenced intestinal contractions, and they showed that the effect of these substances could be neutralized by naloxone. The term they used for the brain's natural opiates was enkephalins, from the Greek for "in the head."

Snyder and his co-workers, independently, used receptor technology to search directly in brain tissue for opiatelike substances. Within a few weeks of the Scottish group, they isolated and purified substances that competed directly with naloxone binding, just as morphine had.

Snyder's team called their substances endorphins, from the words "endogenous morphinelike substances." The two words that describe the brain's natural opiates are used somewhat interchangeably. The two groups of researchers shared the Lasker Award.

In early 1976 scientists at the Salk Institute in San Diego discovered the first of many more endorphins, and pain research was never to be the same.

The impact of these discoveries is hard, even after a decade, to overestimate. Among other things, they may explain how and why acupuncture works. Scientists have found increased levels of endorphins in the blood of individuals undergoing the procedure.

Snyder, Pert, and Michael J. Kuhar, also at Johns Hopkins, have found endorphins in regions of the brain involved not in pain perception, but in emotions. Their findings explain the euphoric — as opposed to the analgesic — powers of narcotics and suggest possible ways to help morphine addicts by blocking those regions of the brain.

The Key to Safer, Better Pain Relief

Most of all, however, these findings opened the door to new strategies in the search for safer, better pain relievers.

The first thought, of course, was whether synthetic endorphins themselves, in a pill form, could fight pain. Because we are clearly not "addicted" to ourselves — the brain's own

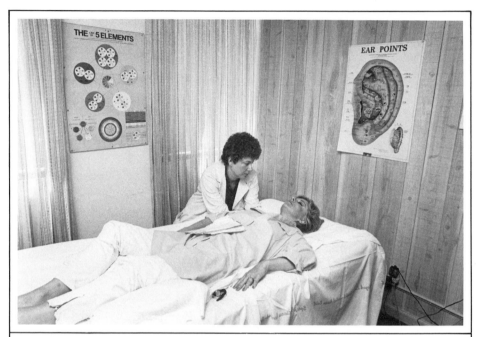

A patient receives acupuncture therapy. Increasingly, medical professionals are recognizing the ancient Oriental technique as a safe and nonaddictive form of pain relief.

morphine is released only at times of extreme pain or stress —it would follow that endorphins are safer than narcotics.

Unfortunately, endorphins break down too quickly and last too briefly to be of real value in the treatment of pain. But manipulation of their chemical structure may produce longer-acting varieties that do work.

Use of endorphinlike products may be superior to anything we now have for treating the pain of diarrhea without side effects in the brain, and several companies are developing such products.

The understanding of painkilling brought about by the discovery of the brain's own opiates has also led to the development of synthetic compounds that may provide new, nonaddictive painkillers. Among these substances are agonist-antagonist mixtures such as pentazocine (Talwin), nalbuphine (Nubain), and butorphanol (Stadol).

Research has shown that some narcotic antagonists have analgesic effects as well. Less addictive than standard natural or synthetic narcotics, these drugs can also be given orally; they do not cause the life-threatening breathing depression that occurs with very high doses of narcotics, and overdosing is less of a risk.

The links forged by nature between pleasure and pain are clearer than ever, and in decades to come scientists are expected to take advantage of those links in their ongoing search for better therapy.

Narcotics — dangerous though they are — have, ironically, taught us much about safer pain relief and about pain itself. Says Snyder: "The opiates have proved to be invaluable tools for investigating how the brain perceives pain and regulates our emotional state. The story of opiate receptors and enkephalins also [will furnish strategies] for the development of new and better [drugs]."

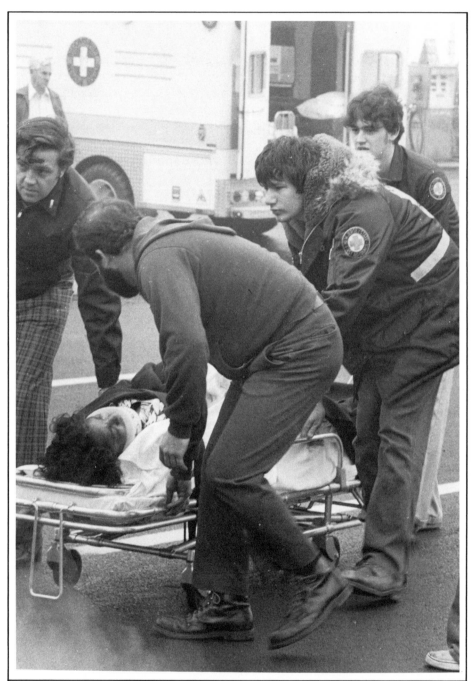

Medical teams must often make life-and-death decisions about which drugs to administer in an emergency, paying special attention to a wide range of potentially dangerous side effects.

CHAPTER 5

SIDE EFFECTS: PSYCHOACTIVE AND OTHERWISE

Suppose you had a headache and a friendly clerk offered you, straight off the supermarket shelf, some pills for the pain that had the following possible side effects: ulcers, severe bleeding, inflammation of mucous membranes, diarrhea, stomach cramps, severe breathing difficulty, skin rashes, shock, asthma, insulin shock, jaundice, kidney damage, ringing in the ears, nausea, blurred vision, mental confusion, vomiting, indigestion, and death.

At the very least, you might think twice about taking the pills or wonder how the drug could be offered without a prescription.

In fact, however, an estimated 30 million Americans — including millions of teenagers — take it each week without a prescription and without thinking twice. We are talking about aspirin.

The above list of side effects associated with aspirin is accurate. Medical scientists half-jokingly note that if the Bayer company's chemists had been forced to seek approval from the FDA to market their wonder drug a century ago, they would have been turned down flat and told aspirin was too dangerous a drug to give people.

But experience and common sense tell us that very few of the millions of people who use aspirin daily will hemorrhage, vomit, or die or in fact suffer any side effects. The point is that *all* painkillers (like all drugs) have side effects. *All* are

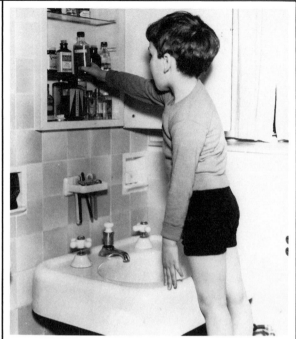

Very young children should never have access to even OTC medicines, and teens and adults alike should read product labels carefully for proper dosage information.

double-edged swords — they may help or hurt. The decision to use a pain reliever should take into account the potential risks as well as the benefits.

Fortunately, drugs sold in the United States must have FDA approval, and their labels must disclose known side effects. Moreover, as it turns out, many of the worst side effects occur only in people with readily identifiable susceptibilities.

In the case of aspirin, for example, studies show that fewer than 1% of the population is allergic to the main ingredient in aspirin — salicylates — and therefore at risk as to skin rashes, breathing problems, or shock. In people with asthma, the rate reaches 5%. Therefore, anyone with a history of asthma is wise to avoid aspirin, particularly for minor or moderate aches and pains that could be handled with simple home remedies or aspirin substitutes.

Similarly, an estimated 5% of those who use aspirin suffer some indigestion, nausea, or other stomach upset from using the substance. These side effects may be offset by "buffering" or drinking milk with the aspirin tablets. People may be willing to risk a bit of indigestion to ease the pain of a torn ligament, but if they already have a history of stomach ulcers, they may not be willing to take the risk.

Increasing the Risk of Side Effects

There are several factors that can influence the likelihood of side effects in narcotics, aspirin, and other painkillers.

Using Drugs in Combination

Drugs used in combination create a new category of potential dangers. The interactions among certain drugs often produce unwanted symptoms and problems that are not a risk when any one of the drugs in question is taken singly.

An example of this point is that both alcohol and salicylates irritate the lining of the digestive tract. Together, they may cause serious stomach upsets or even bleeding in a person who would experience neither symptom with alcohol or aspirin alone. So it is not a good idea to take aspirin for the headache pain of a hangover or to take aspirin with any syrupy medication that may contain alcohol.

People who are taking medication for diabetes, sulfa drugs, tranquilizers, or antidepressants should not take aspirin products. Some people who use PABA — the active ingredient in sunblocks — become overly sensitive to aspirin as well. Many of the risks associated with aspirin apply to the use of acetaminophen as well.

Potency and Site of Action

The stronger a pain reliever is and the longer it is used, the more likely it is to cause undesirable side effects. Narcotic analgesics, such as morphine, work best against severe, deep pain but are also far more likely than nonnarcotic painkillers to create mental confusion, loss of normal brain activity, and interruption of the many chemical "factories" that the brain operates. These drugs also pose a more serious risk of dependency, addiction, and learning and memory deficits than codeine or nonnarcotic analgesics. Drugs that act directly on the brain are more likely to create unpredictable and undesirable side effects than those that do not.

Most people appreciate that the abuse or excessive use of narcotic and other drugs is a guarantee of ill effects. For instance, as mentioned in Chapter 4, the possible side effects of all natural and synthetic narcotics include drowsiness, respiratory depression, nausea, disorientation, increased pulse rate and blood pressure, insomnia, loss of appetite, convulsions, irritability, tremors, chills, sweating, cramps, coma, and death.

Fewer people understand that even when these substances are used for short periods and in mild or moderate dosages, physical, intellectual, and emotional side effects are possible. In one study doctors studied patients who entered a pain treatment center at the Mayo Clinic in Rochester, Minnesota. The study looked at drug use during a three-day period during which the subjects were allowed to give themselves as much or as little of the drugs as they wished. All the subjects were given IQ tests, tests of verbal learning, and memory and personality tests. Results supported the doctors' suspicions that the chronic use of narcotics and tranquilizers, even in moderate dosages, can cause mental and psychological impairment.

The subjects were disorganized, slow, and unable to solve problems, deal with stress, or complete simple tasks. These difficulties were often present even though basic brain and central nervous system functions appeared normal and active.

Pregnancy

Pregnancy is another significant issue in the use of drugs. The sensible rule for girls and women who are pregnant, or might be, is to avoid all drugs unless a physician who knows about the pregnancy or possibility of a pregnancy approves. The reason for this precaution is that there is a whole category of side effects from drugs, including pain relievers, that affect only pregnant women and/or their fetuses. Simple aspirin, for example, can interfere with blood clotting in both the mother and child, lengthen pregnancy and delivery, and increase the incidence of stillbirths and newborn deaths. Narcotic analgesics can induce brain damage, addiction, or death in unborn or newborn babies.

Age

Age is an important factor in susceptibility to the side effects of painkillers. The bodies of infants and children, for example, metabolize and use drugs differently than those of adults, and their central nervous systems and other organs are more vulnerable to certain products. Older people often have

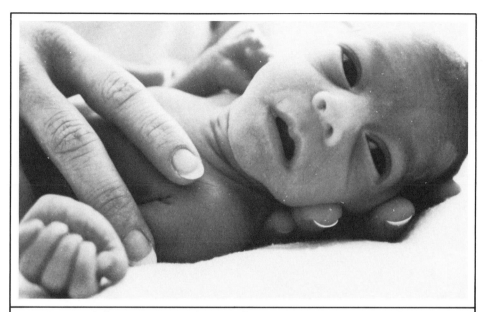

Many painkillers can severely complicate pregnancy and childbirth. Some can lead to premature birth, brain damage, addiction, or death in unborn or newborn infants.

slower metabolisms. In addition, their circulatory systems and the liver and kidneys which play a vital role in ridding the body of drug by-products, may have slowed down as a result of the aging process. In some cases, therefore, a drug may stay too long in an older person's body, increasing the risk of side effects.

Dose

The dosage of certain medications plays a role in determining possible side effects. Many who use pain relievers mistakenly believe that if one or two pills are good, three or four are better, or that if the pain does not go away in 15 or 30 minutes with one dose, they should take another right away. Drug dosages are carefully calculated and take into account body weight, age, and the potency (amount of active ingredients) of the drug.

Moreover, some analgesics — codeine, for example — take a while before they begin to work. Attempts to speed up the process by taking more codeine doses closer together

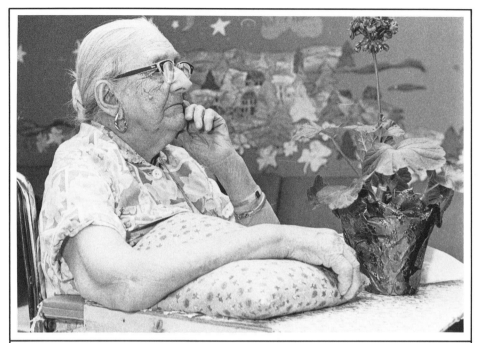

Slower bodily functions in elderly people can affect normal drug absorption. Physicians must consider the age of their patients when prescribing pain relievers and other drugs.

can lead to serious nausea and vomiting. In some cases, doctors will suggest that their patients take aspirin (which acts faster) along with the codeine (which takes longer but works better). This kind of combination treatment must be carefully undertaken to avoid other side effects.

Some products, such as Anacin, advertise that they have "more of the pain reliever doctors prescribe most" (aspirin) and suggest that they are therefore more effective than standard dosage products. However, tests show that products containing 400 mg or more of aspirin per pill compared to the 325 mg in most standard tablets are likely to increase the number and severity of side effects and are *unlikely* to provide any increase in pain relief. More is not always better.

It is extremely important to respect recommended doses in order to avoid side effects, which may range from mild to fatally toxic. Aspirin overdose is the primary cause of death by poisoning among children under five. Excessive use of acetaminophen by people with chronic arthritis or joint pain has been associated with permanent liver damage. If the medicine you are taking does not work in the recommended doses, assume the following: the medicine is the wrong one, or your ailment is not what you think it is. For example, while aspirin is effective in treating the ache of simple muscle strain, it is less so in treating muscular pain caused by a viral infection, such as mononucleosis. It is a rule of thumb that if two tablets of a simple, over-the-counter analgesic such as aspirin, acetaminophen, or ibuprofen do not ease your headache or muscle ache within about 20 or 30 minutes, more will not help.

Adjusting dosages may eliminate unwanted effects of drugs but before decreasing or increasing the dose of any painkiller, consult a physician or pharmacist about the possible consequences.

Sensitivities

Sometimes, of course, patients turn out to have particular sensitivities to a drug or additives used in its preparation. All drugs are chemicals. They are also formulated, or packaged, with fillers, buffers, dyes, and other ingredients, such as alcohol. These added products are often needed to make firm tablets, easy-to-swallow coatings, better-tasting liquids, and so on. Some people are allergic to various chemicals or chemical families as well as to the added products. Patients sometimes discover sensitivities the hard way — by suffering the side effects. Perhaps the most widely publicized is sensitivity to penicillin, an allergy so fierce in some people that taking it will produce anaphylactic shock — a shutdown of the respiratory system—and death.

Some painkillers — among them aspirin — have a history of being more likely to produce sensitivity or allergic reactions, so read labels carefully. Many people are unaware that products such as Alka-Seltzer, Midol, 4-Way Cold Tablets, and Equagesic contain aspirin.

Form and Route of Administration

The form in which painkillers are taken and the way in which they are administered also influence — for some — the risk of side effects. With buffering, aspirin products may not cause upset stomach in many people who get indigestion from the unbuffered product. Drugs injected into the bloodstream work faster than those taken orally. Chewable aspirin and aspirin gum are easy to take and tasty for children but may hurt and irritate any mouth sores they may have.

Timing

The time at which drugs are taken can seriously raise or lower susceptibility to side effects. Some medications should be taken on an empty stomach; others should never be. Some work best if a full day's dose is spread out over several administrations throughout the day, whereas others work better if the full dose is taken all at once or only twice a day.

Long-acting tablets and capsules should be swallowed whole. If chewed, the entire dose of medicine may enter the system all at once, a potentially dangerous situation.

Some medications that ease the torture of migraine headaches work very well if taken at the first subtle sign of an oncoming episode and do nothing at all if the headache is already established.

Recent research has also uncovered the fact that some drugs work faster or slower, better or worse, depending on our body clocks. All living things have a biological "rhythm," a cycle of ups and downs, peaks and valleys, when natural processes and chemicals ebb and flow. The ability of the body to use drugs and the likelihood of side effects is influenced by such timing.

Some General Rules

Appendix II lists many analgesics, both narcotic and nonnarcotic, by brand name, along with suggested uses and side effects to watch out for. In addition, there are several books and guides available in libraries and stores to help you sort out potential side effects and decide whether the risk/benefit ratio benefits you in any decision to take any pain reliever for any particular episode of pain. Among them: the American Pharmaceutical Association's *Handbook of Nonprescription Drugs* and *Evaluations of Drug Interactions*, and the *Physicians' Desk Reference*.

But there are some general rules that can protect you and help you avoid side effects:

• *Never* take someone else's prescription pain relievers, even if you believe you have the same symptoms from the same cause. Prescription drugs are tailored — in content, dose, and directions for use — to the individual patient. Another user may not be aware of all the possible ill effects or risky drug interactions.

• Read labels for active ingredients and additional ingredients to which you may be allergic. A tip: if a close relative (parent, brother, sister) is sensitive to a drug, you are likely to be as well.

• For nonprescription pain relievers, you can often rely on a registered pharmacist who either knows or can look up on the spot the side effects of particular pain relievers. There is no charge for this service.

• *Never* take a pain reliever without a doctor's advice if you are also taking any prescription drugs, have any diseases, are pregnant or nursing, or if your symptoms have lasted longer than a week to 10 days. You need professional medical advice.

• Avoid the use of combination products that contain two or more active ingredients. The reason: it is hard to determine what is to blame if you have a bad side effect. Single-ingredient products reduce the risk of poisoning, allergic reactions, and other problems.

• Do not buy *any* medication that does not list the names and amounts of its ingredients.

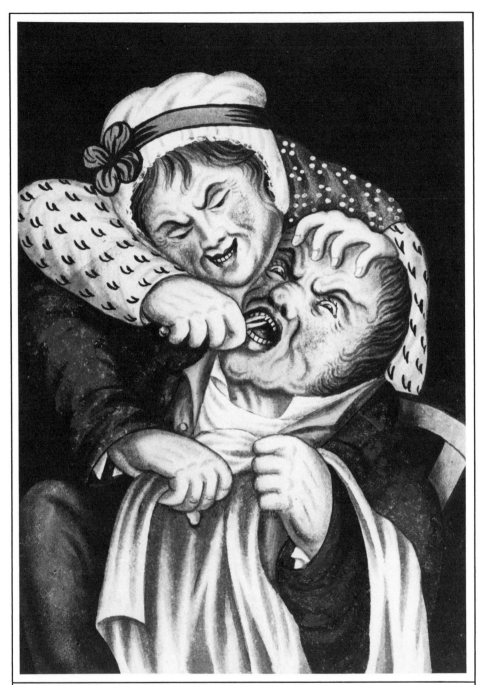

A grimly comic drawing captures the terror that pain in all its guises holds for most people. The anticipation of pain can make it even worse; relaxation techniques can minimize these anxieties.

CHAPTER 6

ASSESSING YOUR PAIN: HOW MUCH DOES IT HURT?

Drew: I can't make it to school this morning. My head and throat are killing me.

Mom: I'm sure it hurts, but I've had colds before, too. Just take a couple of aspirin and you'll feel good enough to make it to class.

Drew (*angrily*): This isn't just an ordinary cold. The pain is much worse. I ought to know. I'm the one feeling it.

Every teenager who has had this conversation (is there one who has not?) has a clue to the problem of assessing pain. How much does it *really* hurt? Enough to stay home from school? To need a doctor's attention? Aspirin? Narcotics? And, perhaps most important of all, what does the pain mean? Is it "just a cold"? Or does the pain signal something more serious? What if it is really serious and no one believes it is? Or what if it is serious and no one can find out why? Is that pain in your side gas? Or appendicitis? Is that headache a migraine? A brain tumor? Or just a muscle-tension headache?

Obviously, answers to those questions have more serious implications than convincing Mom to let you stay home for the day. Each of us must learn to evaluate and "read" the ordinary and not-so-ordinary aches and pains that we experience. How well we do it may determine not only how safely and effectively we manage our bouts of pain — with drugs or without — but also how well we manage our lives and health.

The world is heartily unsympathetic to people who are "always complaining," "always in pain," or disabled by dubious miseries. "Scratch a hypochondriac," says a psychiatrist who treats adults with this disorder, "and you'll often find someone who never learned to understand what all the assorted aches and pains everyone has when they were kids really meant. *Everything* took on equal importance, until everything became an equal threat."

Needless to say, the issue is not whether to ignore or pay attention to pain. All pain is a signal of some sort of problem. The issue is to sort out pain that is a symptom of a condition that poses serious harm from pain that is self-limiting, a symptom of a temporary and minor upset in the delicate balance of operations that keeps us going.

It is possible to learn to assess your own pain. The results help not only to find the right "home remedy" if that is in order but also to help parents and physicians understand your pain and find safe, effective relief.

Whenever teenagers hurt, they might find it reassuring to keep these facts in mind:

• Adolescence is a time of rapid mental and physical growth and of many changes. These occurrences conspire at times to trigger pains, some never experienced before and some more intense or frequent than experienced in the past. In short, as one grows and matures, pain is to be *expected*.

Adults often — mistakenly — believe that children and adolescents who are physically and mentally healthy should have little or no pain. The fact is that numerous studies show that young people are *more* likely to experience pain such as headaches, backaches, muscle pains, stomach pains, premenstrual and menstrual cramps, and dental pain than are older people.

"Growing pains" are real enough. Although it is true that they eventually go away by themselves, they still need attention and sometimes treatment. During the growth spurts that occur periodically in adolescence, tendons and joints may be stretched and stressed. Until hormone changes stabilize, the body's natural chemicals can contract and dilate blood vessels that trigger migraines and cramps.

• Pain is not necessarily evil. In fact, pain is truly, at times, a friend. It can save lives. As the body's alarm system, it tells

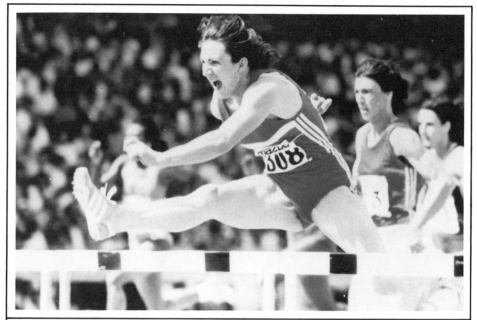

Like professional athletes, active teenagers are strong candidates for sports injuries. In addition, hormonal levels change profoundly during adolescence and this, too, may cause discomfort.

us something is hurting us, gets us to stop moving so as not to aggravate the injury, and gives us time to heal. Experts are not suggesting that people should be grateful for pain, but they are aware of the disastrous consequences that come from the inability to feel pain.

There is, for example, an extremely rare genetic disease whose victims lack normal pain-nerve pathways. For these people, the world is a painless agony. Their fingers are crushed and burned by doors and flames they cannot feel. They are permanently deformed by dislocated and broken bones caused by accidents they cannot feel and therefore cannot learn to avoid. Their joints are damaged by overexertion. Deep ulcers and cuts occur because they cannot feel sharp objects as they crawl or play.

• Suppressing pain can be a dangerous trap. Sometimes it is important to let pain emerge so that you and your physician can tell where it is coming from, how intense it is, and what the signal really means.

A zealous cheerleader outshouted her entire squad at a Saturday football game and developed a sore throat that evening. She began at once to take two aspirins, then three, every three or four hours. By Sunday night the pain was worse, so she added gargles and lozenges. By midweek she agreed to let her doctor take a throat culture, and the lab reported a "strep" (streptococcal bacteria) infection. What she needed were antibiotics. Her efforts to mask her pain had allowed her to mistake a serious illness — strep — for the temporary distress of vocal cord strain.

Untreated strep infections can be dangerous and may even damage the heart. In this case, fortunately, the only damage was five unnecessary days of suffering. The mild throat irritation that comes from a few hours of shouting usually goes away by itself after a few hours of silence and some soothing drinks. That early aspirin treatment dulled the pain signals just enough in the early stages to fool the cheerleader and her family.

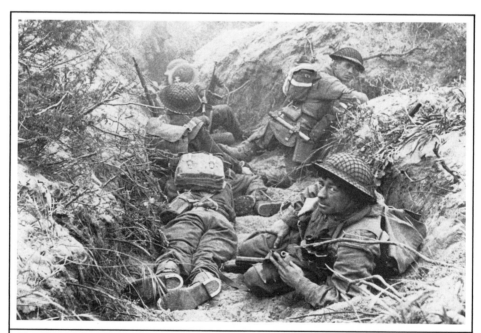

The "Anzio" effect illustrates the psychology of pain. Wounded soldiers in this battle knew their injuries meant an escape from war and therefore suffered less than civilians with similar injuries.

• Because fear and uncertainty play so large a role in pain and how it is perceived, teenagers should let those who care about them know if they are in pain. Often those with more experience handling pain can be instantly reassuring.

For example, a young girl experiencing her first menstrual cramps may become tense with fear, aggravating the pain, unless she understands what the pain means.

In another case, an older teenager, unaccustomed to physical inactivity after being ill with infectious mononucleosis, was stunned and frightened at the amount of muscle pain he felt after he resumed jogging. He did not understand that it takes months to become fit and only days or weeks to lose the edge. The pain was his body's way of saying, "Slow down and take this carefully."

Another teenage athlete withheld from his parents and coach for days the fact that he found it painful to urinate. When he finally consulted his physician, the condition was diagnosed as a noninfectious inflammation, possibly caused by an injury. Some warm baths solved the problem.

• What pain means often determines how people react to it. According to Raymond Houde, a pain-drug research expert at New York's Memorial Sloan-Kettering Cancer Center, stress, anxiety, and expectations can make pain seem more severe. He found, for example, that patients who had been successfully treated for cancer would sometimes find a simple stomach ache excruciating because of the fear that the pain signaled a return of their disease.

This link between pain and its meaning for any individual is dramatically shown in what is called the "Anzio" effect. Anzio, Italy, was the site of a particularly bloody battle during World War II. Pain scientist Henry Beecher found that soldiers at Anzio who were wounded in the chest or abdomen needed far less morphine to control pain than civilians who had experienced surgery or injuries that created identical wounds. The explanation turned out to be simple: for the civilians the wounds and pain were a source of anxiety. For the soldiers the wounds and pain meant they were going home and were out of the fearful war for good.

• Some people are more susceptible to *chronic* pain than others. Acute pain, the kind that occurs quickly, is often intense but goes away rapidly. Chronic pain recurs and stays

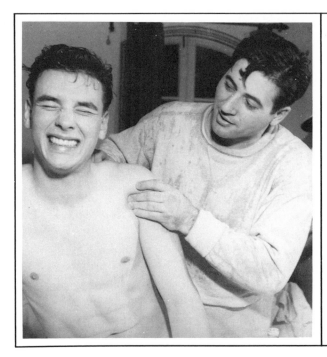

A pitcher receives a rubdown after the first workout of a season. Even professional athletes can lose muscle tone quickly if regular exercise is neglected; reconditioning these muscles once they become flabby is difficult and often painful. Fortunately, massage can help relieve muscular aches.

around, coming and going in an often unpredictable fashion and creating a cycle of pain and anticipation of pain that makes people feel helpless and unable to control their lives.

Scientists have evidence that people who lack motivation, self-esteem, and pride in their achievements and those who are dependent on others are more likely to experience chronic pain than those who are highly motivated to get on with their lives and be independent.

• There is a strong psychological component to pain. The so-called placebo (Latin for "I will please") effect is a case in point. Scientists at the University of California in San Francisco reported that a sugar pill designed to look like various drugs produced the effect of mild doses of morphine if patients truly believed the pill would work.

But parents, teachers, or physicians who use such evidence to dismiss a complaint of pain as "being all in your head" or claim to "prove the case" by pointing out that distractions make the pain go away are often not aware of the real problem.

Joan (*leaving for field hockey practice*): I'll see you later.

Dad: What happened to the terrible headache you had a little while ago when it was time to clean up the kitchen?

Joan: The team needs me. Anyway, I feel a little better.

Dad may be right. Joan's perception of her pain can be influenced by motivation. On the other hand, that does not mean her pain was not real when the dishes were piled in the sink with the breakfast eggs stuck to them.

According to many studies, fewer than 5% of chronic-pain patients are hypochondriacs. Pain — not the perception of pain—is what makes most people suffer in the first place.

• Pain is often not remembered accurately or at all. In a recent Canadian study, 25 "tension" headache patients kept a daily pain diary, writing down each hour the intensity of the pain they felt. At each office visit they also rated the intensity of the pain they felt at the moment and were asked to recall how it compared to what their between-visit headaches felt like.

The scientists found that when the current pain was bad, the patients tended to "remember" their past headaches as worse than they actually were (as recorded in the diary). When current pain was low, they recalled past pain as less severe than they had recorded it.

Pain, the scientists concluded, distorts our memory of pain. Acute pain is often not remembered at all. Many have observed that if we did remember it, no woman would have more than one child.

Measuring Pain

Most of the pains suffered by normal, healthy teenagers are likely to be short-lived and easily handled with rest, heat, ice, and minor medications. Different people respond differently to the same pain, depending on their physical development, the context in which the pain is felt, what the pain means for them, and how the people around them react to their pain.

How, then, if there is no standard of pain, can pain be accurately measured?

Scientists have developed a number of ways to measure physical pain apart from the psychological factors that influence it. One purpose is to have an objective way to evaluate how well drugs work against particular kinds of pain.

In the 1950s dolorologists (literally, students of pain) used devices such as pressure gauges applied to the forehead to try to establish a standard pain threshold — the precise moment when a stimulus produced discomfort. The gauge assigned a number value to the subject's pain response, ranging from none to agony. The problem with these devices was that they did not take into account biochemical or psychological differences that made some individuals more or less able to ignore or tolerate pain at lower levels.

Other methods measured pain tolerance (the most intense stimulation people can endure) or used scales in which patients were given a set number of categories (mild, moderate, severe) and asked to rate their pain.

These methods rarely have any relationship to the real, clinical pain people claim to suffer. Most recent techniques, therefore, have focused on complicated visual scales, in which patients are asked to indicate the magnitude of their pain along a straight line. In these tests, the patients compare the intensity of one painful stimulus to another using their eyes.

Taking Charge

Most of us, however, do not need complicated routines to assess everyday pain. Here are some questions to ask yourself to help assess your pain and tell you which steps to take and when to take them.

• Can you explain the pain? An easy case: the person who wakes up with a splitting headache and drank too much the night before is not likely to worry about a brain tumor. Other cases seem tougher but if you think hard are just as easily explained. Imagine a teenager who wakes up with an excruciating, nerve-jangling, immobilizing pain radiating down his neck to his right shoulder and arm. He calls for strong medicine, convinced that morphine, at the very least, should be administered.

The prospect of a stroke, nerve damage, and other dire problems loom in his tortured imagination. Then his mother, who works for an orthopedic surgeon and knows a little about nerves, muscles, and teenagers, reminds him of his activities the night before. He had been talking for hours on the telephone with the receiver alternately nestled in the crook of his neck or held in his right hand with his elbow propped up on a table. His neck and shoulder simply had a giant spasm. Massage, heat, and a day off the telephone cure the pain.

Try to recall a forgotten bump or fall or a new exercise that cramped or pulled your muscles. Perhaps a recent illness or injury has flared up again. In many cases the source of the pain may be tracked to something transient and minor. Relief may require nothing more than a little time, some rest, a couple of aspirin, acetaminophen, or ibuprofen tablets, and perhaps heat or cold or massage.

• Have you had a good checkup lately? If you have more than occasional bouts of pain, a checkup (physical and dental) can rule out such causes as chronic infections, anemia and other nutritional problems, allergic conditions that trigger sinus and headache pain, problems with posture and bone development, impacted teeth, jaw misalignment, or a hidden injury.

It is often difficult, but nonetheless important, to describe specifically the nature and longevity of pain to a doctor so that he or she can properly diagnose and treat it.

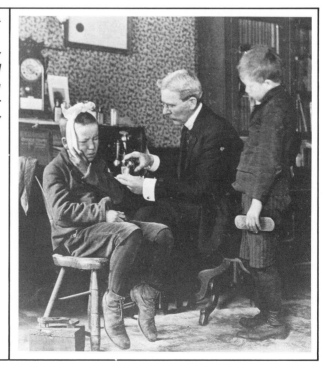

• Is there a pattern to the pain? Does it come and go in a predictable way? Menstrual and premenstrual pain is one example of regular, predictable pain. Muscle soreness after heavy workouts on the Monday after a lazy weekend is another. The reason to pay attention to patterns is to be aware of when the pattern shifts or the pain becomes far more intense than is usual. If that muscle soreness on Monday is suddenly disabling, you may have an injury that needs attention. If headaches suddenly begin to occur every day after school, you may need eyeglasses or a change of prescription.

• Is your pain a type you have *never* experienced before? A brand-new kind of pain, if it stays more than a little while and is intense, should be reported and checked out.

• Do you have other symptoms with your pain? Fever? Nausea? When pain is accompanied by other symptoms the chances are increased that there is an infection or injury that needs attention. Do not cover up the symptoms with medications, especially if the pain has lasted a day or two. Pain of this kind needs to be checked out by a doctor.

• Is the pain stopping you from doing what you normally do? What you want to do? Any pain that does this, whether you think it is caused by something serious or not, needs to be investigated. Unless the pain is a result of a serious underlying disease or major injury, a combination of drugs, rest, physical therapy, and other treatments can almost always restore the ability to get back into your most important activities.

• Can you quickly and easily make the pain go away? If you can — through relaxation, for example, or two aspirin — make occasional headaches or body aches go away within a half hour, the chances are excellent the pain is "benign." It is unlikely to cause you any lasting problems or harm.

• Are you under an unusual amount of stress? Everyone experiences stress in daily life, but at certain times — final exams, term-paper deadlines, a divorce in your family, romantic problems — stress is exceptionally bad. Pains that are at other times tolerable may become intolerable when stress levels are very high. Just being aware of the situation and knowing that the high-stress period may soon ease up can lessen the pain and help you put it in perspective.

• How intense is the pain? How long a pain lasts and its magnitude are important parts of pain assessment. A headache or backache that lasts a whole day and is not relieved at least in part by simple analgesics within a half hour of taking them may be a signal of illness or injury that needs watching. Pain that lasts more than a few days — anywhere in the body — needs to be checked out.

• How can you get the message that you are in pain across to parents and doctors? Whining and complaining in vague terms rarely work. If you have a pain that is worrying you, tell someone, as precisely as you can, where it hurts and why you think it hurts. If you cannot track down a source, a pain diary may help reveal a pattern. In the diary, try to rate the pain in contrast to other pain you have had. Keep a daily record of when the pain seems to be better or worse, what seems to aggravate or ease it, and what pain relievers or other remedies you have tried to relieve it. Specific information will help others understand and find the right treatment faster.

• What does the pain mean to you? This is the hardest question for most of us to answer honestly and objectively, but an objective answer can put you on the road to relief.

The daughter of a doctor began to suffer terrible headache pain when her father was about to retire. She was able to reduce the frequency and severity of the headaches when she faced the fact that she was very worried about her father's ability to adapt to retirement. Her pain was one possible way of giving him a perpetual patient! Do you sometimes have pain that gets you sympathy, helps others feel important or needed, or gives you a breather in an "impossible" schedule? Then you are in good company. Understanding the psychological, emotional, or interpersonal function such pain is playing in your life may start you on the road not only to pain relief but also to some long-term solutions to problems that may be disrupting your life.

———————◇———————

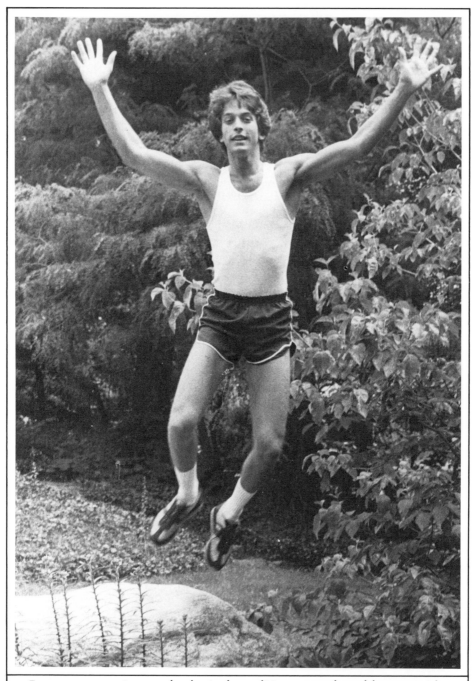

Even teenagers in superb physical condition are vulnerable to a wide variety of aches and pains. Often, however, these discomforts do not require drug therapy and clear up on their own within days.

CHAPTER 7

WHERE DOES IT HURT? TEENAGE PAINS

Where does a teenager hurt?

Anywhere a person can.

Tender age is no barrier to a painful existence or guarantor of a painless one. Indeed, young people are especially *prone* to headaches, backaches, muscle pains, stomach pains, toothaches, and menstrual pain. The only major categories of pain found more frequently in older people are those associated with arthritis and such older age-linked diseases as cancer, heart disease, and diabetes.

Whatever the cause and wherever it strikes, pain kidnaps your attention, driving you in search of peace and, too often, chemical ransom. That goes for teenagers no less than adults.

What follows is a compendium of common pains and what typically causes them. Not a single one of them is "imaginary" or "all in the head."

Keep in mind, however, that many teenage pains are what physicians call "self-limiting," meaning they will go away without drugs and usually in a matter of hours or days. Drugs may be useful to make you more comfortable and help you rest while your body heals and pain nerves settle down.

Headaches

Headaches are the number-one pain problem of all time. Children were once thought to be relatively immune to headaches, but more recent surveys strongly suggest that 20% of American children have migraine or serious tension headaches, and 40% of all migraine victims have their first episode before the age of 15.

Scientists do not always agree on what causes a headache. Everything from weather and allergies to air pollution, menstruation, oversleeping, and even bright light are to blame for some headaches.

For teenagers, a combination of hereditary factors, personality, and social factors is often the cause of a headache. Migraine victims, for example, do seem to inherit bodies and chemistries that are especially vulnerable, possibly because they were born with blood vessels that are unusually "plastic" and dilate easily. But even with a hereditary ailment the pain does not arrive without a trigger such as stress or a change in air pressure.

There are four major types of headache. Muscle-contraction headaches, popularly known as tension headaches, are the most common by far and can usually be eased with relaxation. Vascular headaches, caused by swollen blood vessels, include migraines. Teenagers and even children can and do get minor vascular headaches, especially so-called ice-cream headaches, which occur after rapidly eating very cold foods. Secondary headaches are those caused by disease or injuries to the head. These are rare but require fast medical treatment. Finally, there are the very rare psychological and "conversion" headaches triggered entirely by stress.

Studies suggest that less than 25% of all headaches need professional medical help and less than 2% are due to serious physical ailments, such as a tumor or sinus infection.

When you have a headache, play detective. Do the pains come only at certain times, such as after exercising? Only when you wake up or on weekends? Do you clench your teeth a lot or read in bad light? Is it almost time for your period?

If your headache feels like a bank of pressure on both sides of your head and is frequent, you probably have the muscle-tension variety. If it is around the temple and forehead, simple eye strain is a likely cause.

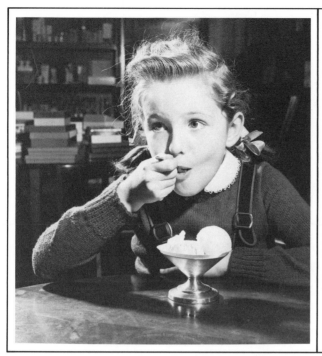

Gulping down ice cream and other cold foods can bring on a headache. These pains are not muscular — they result from a swelling of blood vessels in the head.

Migraines are marked by pain on one side of the head, throbbing, and nausea. They may also be accompanied by visual "auras" or the perception of unusual odors half an hour or less before the pain begins. Chances are good a member of your immediate family has them as well.

Menstrual headaches have the same root causes as migraine—swelling of blood vessels in the head.

Headache treatments include not only relaxation but also simple analgesics (for muscle tension headaches), muscle relaxers, tranquilizers, special drugs that help contract blood vessels, and diets that remove foods that are linked to headaches in some people.

Watch out with drugs, however. According to recent studies, long-term, frequent use of codeine, Demerol, or even aspirin may actually make headaches worse by overloading biochemical receptors in the brain. A study at the New England Center for Headache in Greenwich, Connecticut, for example, found that a month after patients were taken off painkillers, two-thirds reported that they suffered fewer headaches than when they were taking the medications. When it comes to aspirin, if two do not relieve your headache in thirty minutes, no amount will.

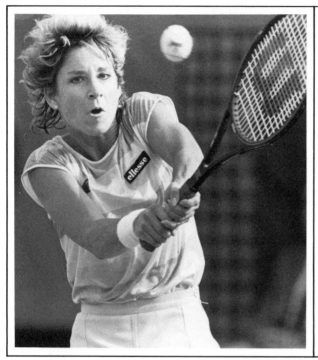

Professional tennis stars, such as Chris Evert Lloyd, are especially vulnerable to the pains of "tennis elbow," characterized by swelling in the elbow region and possible ligament injury.

Low-Back Pain

Most low-back pain is the price we pay for walking upright and for not getting enough exercise. For females, high-heeled shoes that interfere with posture are villains as well. The upright position puts pressure on the spongy, round shock-absorbing discs located in the lower end of the back. Poor posture and disuse of the muscles that brace the spine contribute to pain. Sitting hunched over a desk, standing on your feet all day, lifting, and bending are sure ways to suffer stiffness and dull ache.

The best "cure" is prevention. Keeping the muscles around the spine fit, bending at the knees instead of at the waist, and maintaining good posture are all good insurance against low-back pain. Teenagers who sprawl in the easy chair to do homework, sleep on oversoft mattresses, or slump over their school desks increase their risk of low-back pain.

Once afflicted, most victims of low-back pain find relief in special stretching exercises, heat, and rest. Analgesics are useful at the peak of an attack.

Other Joint and Muscle Pain

Tennis elbow and "cricks" in the neck, stabbing pains in the heel and shin splints are the marks of the joint, tendon, and muscle problems many teenagers experience. Most of these ailments are a consequence of sports injuries and improper training.

Neck pain in the morning may be due to poor sleeping habits — too-soft pillows and mattresses. It may also be a symptom of flu when accompanied by fever and overall achiness.

Pain in the shoulders is common; in fact, there is often an epidemic of this complaint after the first snowfall of a season, when young people are pressed into service to shovel walks and driveways. Playing racquet sports, throwing a football, pitching a baseball, and similar activities are also frequent causes.

The major symptom of tennis elbow is a swelling in the elbow area and sometimes injury to ligaments that bind joints and muscles. The ailments are caused by rolling or twisting motions of the forearm, wrist, and hand and are not only caused by playing tennis.

Runners, joggers, and other track-and-field athletes are prone to damaged tendons, muscles, and ligaments in the feet, heels, and shins.

Rest, ice, aspirin, ibuprofen, steroid (usually cortisone) injections, heat, and — after healing — strength-building exercises are all useful in controlling these pains. In most cases, several days' rest and home remedies are all that are necessary. If the pain, swelling, or tenderness does not begin to subside within a day or two, professional medical help is in order.

Stomach and Abdominal Pains

For most teenagers, stomach and abdominal pains are a source of embarrassment as well as anxiety. Most people do not like to talk about or admit to heartburn, constipation, hemorrhoids, and gas.

Luckily very few abdominal pains are marks of appendicitis. Start to worry only if the pain begins around the navel or below the breastbone and moves to focus on the right lower quarter of the abdomen; if the pain is accompanied by nausea, vomiting, or loss of appetite; if there is local tenderness in the lower right abdomen; and if there is fever.

Diet has a profound influence on many digestive-system problems and the pain they produce, especially heartburn, gas, and constipation. Smoking cigarettes, drinking coffee, tea, alcohol, or milk, and taking aspirin can all cause heartburn and gas. Reclining after a heavy meal, wearing tight-fitting clothes, and eating late-night snacks can lead to gastrointestinal distress.

Eating high-fiber foods, such as salads and bran, can relieve constipation and hemorrhoids. Taken in moderation, mild laxatives are usually safe and effective. (Pain relievers can often upset an already nervous stomach.) Antacids and occasional use of Alka-Seltzer (which has aspirin in it) bring rapid relief of heartburn and nausea to many.

Premenstrual and Menstrual Pains

It is safe to say that no other form of female pain has been the subject of more confusion and bad information than the pain linked to the menstrual cycle.

Every woman experiences the cycle differently, but 40% of all women — especially young women and teenagers — experience this kind of pain. For some, the pain is mild. For others it is crippling pain that lasts hours or days.

Contemporary physicians recognize a pattern of aches, pains, and nervousness, known as premenstrual syndrome or PMS, in the days before menstrual flow begins. Cramps, abdominal tenderness, and headaches during the flow are associated with the release of certain hormones.

The good news for the many thousands who truly suffer from menstrual distress is that there is medication available to treat the problem safely and effectively: over-the-counter and prescription strength ibuprofen. Aspirin, too, is often effective in milder cases.

Dental Pains

Braces — and all the fittings, adjustments, and other procedures that go with them — produce aches, bruises, cuts, irritations, and sometimes serious pain in the mouth and head. Wisdom teeth that are impacted — without room to emerge in the mouth — and gingivitis (an infection of the gums) also plague teenagers.

In most cases pain associated with braces is best handled with mouth rinses and nonprescription analgesics. When the pain is serious, the dentist will often write a prescription for codeine or a similar product.

For impacted wisdom teeth, the safest and best way out of the pain is extraction. The pain after they are pulled may be severe and require narcotics for relief. But these effects last only a day or two, and healing is completed in a few weeks.

Pain of Infections

Viral, bacterial, and fungal infections not only produce fever, fatigue, itching, rashes, blisters, and discharges but also pain. The pain can be anywhere and everywhere — in the head, on the skin, in the glands and sinus cavities, in the throat, nose, and mouth, and deep inside the internal organs.

The important thing to remember about such ailments is that although pain relievers are sometimes useful for temporary relief, they do nothing to treat the underlying infection. Moreover, painkillers may mask the disease, giving it a stronger grip on your system.

Headaches that accompany a common cold or flu can be treated with nonprescription pain relievers, but if that "cold" or "flu" has not begun to fade in a few days, see your doctor.

Pain accompanied by rashes, blisters, burning sensations, discharges from the urinary tract or genital area, bleeding, difficulty breathing, or intense itching need prompt medical attention.

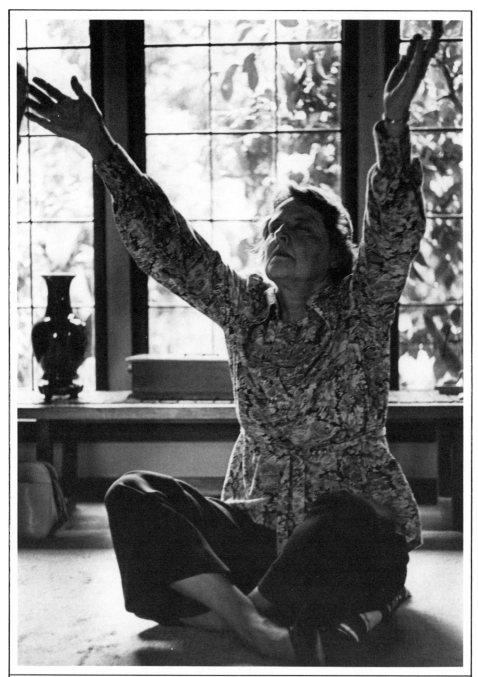

Many people discover that they can relieve pain, partially or completely, by mastering meditative techniques that encourage relaxation and marshal inner psychological strength.

CHAPTER 8

PAIN RELIEF WITHOUT DRUGS

Anyone who has rubbed away the pain of a stubbed toe, massaged a headache into submission, or stopped the pain of an injection by slapping or pinching the entry point first has experimented—successfully—with nondrug pain relief.

Until recently, however, such physical treatments, which also include the use of heat, cold, acupuncture, and electrical stimulation, were generally suspect. Along with psychological therapies such as hypnosis, biofeedback, relaxation, and behavior modification, they were lumped in the category of "mind over matter" and often attacked as quackery or old wives' tales.

New discoveries about the transmission and control of pain, however, are winning respect for these physical and psychological pain remedies. Their biggest advantage over drugs and surgery — total safety and lack of side effects — is focusing increased attention on their use.

Among these discoveries is the brain's own opiate system (see Chapter 4). Scientists are finding that the stress-induced release of endorphins can in fact relieve the pain of injuries such as war wounds.

In the case of rubbing the sore toe, scientists Ronald Melzack and Patrick Wall devised a theory to explain this effect, called the gate-control theory of pain.

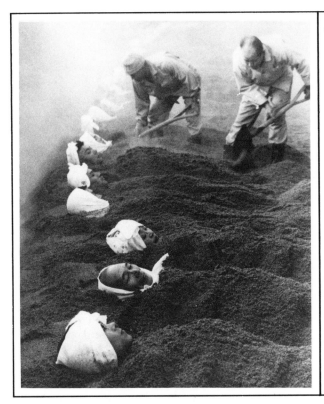

Japanese patients seek relief in sand baths. Many scientists believe that heat applied to the skin overlying a major nerve raises the pain threshold.

The theory says that the pathways along which sensory nerve signals travel can handle only so much traffic at one time. *Any* sensory signal — pain, pressure, itch, tickle, etc. — has equal access to the road. When too many signals are traveling in the system, cells in the spinal column interrupt and close the "gate," stopping all transmission in a kind of neuronal gridlock.

Therefore, when pain signals are coursing along after a person has stubbed a toe, vigorous rubbing overloads the sensory roads and closes the gate to *all* sensation — including the pain. It is why slapping an itch stops the itch.

Working with the idea that applying a "counterirritant" such as rubbing can sabotage the pain transmission network, pain specialists developed TENS, or transcutaneous electric nerve stimulation.

In TENS, electrodes attached to the skin above a painful area send a safe, mild electrical current into the body to compete with the pain-nerve signals and close the gate. Acupuncture treatment (placing needles in selected spots to stimulate nerves under the skin) is believed to bring temporary analgesia by shutting the same gate. In the People's Republic of China many visitors have observed painless surgery performed on conscious patients. The only painkillers used in these operations have been acupuncture needles and small doses of Valium. Some studies suggest that acupuncture may also release endorphins.

According to a report from the National Institutes of Health, evidence from such painless surgery cases suggests that the painlessness is a "result of activation of intrinsic brain mechanisms which profoundly modify the central pattern of nerve impulses necessary to experience pain."

Studies show that TENS brings short-term relief for as many as 80% of all patients, and one-third obtain long-term relief with devices that cost between $60 and $400.

Treatment without drugs can be especially useful for teenagers in pain. Most of these treatments can be done anywhere, with little or no equipment. They leave the mind clear and the body clean. In some cases, one or more such techniques can be combined with drugs to bring pain relief better than any one treatment alone, and often with lower doses of medication.

Here are brief descriptions of some other increasingly popular and scientifically proven nondrug means of pain relief.

Heat and Cold

Studies suggest that the success of therapy using heat and cold is probably best explained by the gate-control theory of pain. Both heat and cold influence receptors or interact with other nerve impulses traveling in the spinal cord or lower portion of the brain.

Physicians have found that heat applied to the skin overlying a major nerve raises the pain threshold. For chronic pain, intense heat is best; for acute pain, milder temperatures are better.

Heat can be applied either on the surface or deeply. Many teenage girls have used heating pads to relieve menstrual cramps—an example of superficial or on-the-surface heat.

Hydrocollators (chemical heat packs) and hot baths are often used by athletes to relieve muscle pain. Deep-heat therapy can be given using ultrasound or microwave radiation, but these require special equipment and medical training.

Cooling the body's surface also elevates the pain threshold and has the added benefit of reducing pain-producing swelling.

If you use heat or cold, be careful to protect the skin from damage.

Exercise

Exercise is one of the most successful but least-used pain control methods. There are specific activities designed to flex and strengthen muscles, stretch the spine, and relieve pressure. It is important to make sure that the exercises are properly performed and will not further injure muscles, tendons, or joints. Numerous studies now confirm that inactivity is a pain producer, not a healer, for a large number of bone, muscle, and joint disorders.

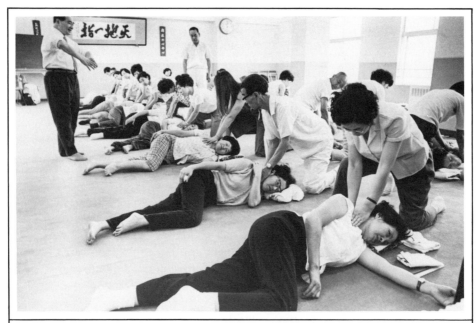

A "Shiatsu" massage can be tremendously effective in relieving several kinds of physical pain and in mentally relaxing the patient.

Massage

Massage is a sort of "passive" exercise. Squeezing, stroking, and rubbing painful areas feels wonderful and can relieve sore, aching muscles and joints. Many people also believe that spinal manipulation, performed by chiropractors and other nonmedical practitioners, relieve back, neck, and other kinds of pain. A workshop sponsored by the National Institute of Neurological and Communicative Disorders and Stroke recently concluded, however, that there is no evidence to prove or disprove the value of spinal manipulation. As a result, most physicians are reluctant to perform or recommend it.

Behavioral Therapy

Behavior is anything we learn to do, including some of our responses to pain. We learn our pain behaviors the way we learn everything else — from our culture, our relatives, our friends, the context in which the pain is suffered, and the attentions and concern of others when pain is a problem. Sometimes these "outside" factors act as "reinforcers" of pain, encouraging us to continue pain behaviors long after the original cause of the pain is under control.

When carried out by psychologists, psychiatrists, and other behavior specialists, behavioral therapy — or behavior modification, as it is also called — successfully attacks pain behaviors that are learned and can therefore be "unlearned." The goal of behavioral therapy is to treat the way we respond to pain or to modify our perception of pain.

Behavioral therapy is often used in combination with drugs and physical therapy. Therapists first evaluate each patient and his or her environment carefully to see what factors are reinforcing pain behavior and how best to interrupt them. The treatment usually includes a step-by-step program for increasing "well" behaviors, such as physical activity; decreasing drug-taking and other pain behaviors; and helping family and friends become aware of how they encourage or discourage pain behavior. These techniques help patients pay more attention to what they *can* do and less attention to what they cannot. They restore and reinforce pain patients' sense of control over themselves.

So powerful are these techniques in the hands of well-trained specialists that even patients with terminal-cancer pain have been able to do without high doses of narcotics.

One of the most powerful aspects of behavior modification is its ability to alter pain perception. Studies have shown that some people anticipate and expect pain while others do not or do so to a lesser extent. The difference is accounted for by what they learn from people around them.

Years ago, this writer witnessed firsthand the effects of learned behavior and expectations on pain perception when my then-three-year-old son was hospitalized for a minor operation.

The surgeon advised me not to offer my son aspirin or other painkillers after the operation unless he clearly showed or complained of pain. He instructed me not to make a big fuss about pain, to look upset and sad, or say things like "Where does it hurt, you poor baby?"

To my surprise my son woke up from his anesthesia, went home several hours later, went straight to sleep, and woke up the next morning without a whimper or an aspirin.

His stitches pulled and he walked a little bent over for a day or so, but that was it.

"Maybe you were surprised, but I'm not," the surgeon said when I told him the story. "He didn't have a chance to learn how to complain a lot and get a lot of attention for having a bit of pain. Make no mistake, he had some discomfort. But if you had invited complaints and made a big fuss about them, you can bet he would have cried, needed pain relievers, and taken a lot longer to get back on his feet and into action."

Biofeedback and Hypnosis

Biofeedback treatment teaches pain patients to be aware of subtle biological changes — such as an increase in blood pressure or contractions in neck muscles. Patients learn this awareness with the help of electronic devices that give visual or audio signals, or feedback, about a body function that is not normally under conscious control. For example, electronic sensors that detect changes in skin temperature are translated into images on a television monitor. The degree of brightness on the screen correlates with increases or decreases in skin temperature.

By sitting and experiencing these connected reactions, patients learn to exercise some control over these body functions and often to reverse the biological mechanisms that cause pain.

For example, for patients with tension headache, electrical activity in neck muscles is monitored and converted, via electrodes, into "clicks." The clicks become more frequent when muscle contraction increases. The patient tries to reduce the clicks by reducing neck-muscle activity. Several studies have found that some patients can learn to control the muscle activity and stop headaches from starting.

Hypnosis is a method that increases a person's susceptibility to suggestion. Studies indicate that hypnosis can bring pain relief in 15% to 20% of selected patients. Hypnotherapy should be performed only by trained and licensed specialists.

Relaxation and Meditation

Relaxation therapy can relieve tension headaches by unknotting muscles associated with head pain, particularly the trapezius, which connects the shoulder blade to the collar and neck bones. Techniques for relaxing these muscles range from hot baths and gentle massage to special muscle exercises. Alternately tensing and relaxing various muscles in regular patterns every day helps patients master the technique so that they can use it when pain strikes.

Meditation refers to techniques that help people relax by blotting out distractions, noise, and worries.

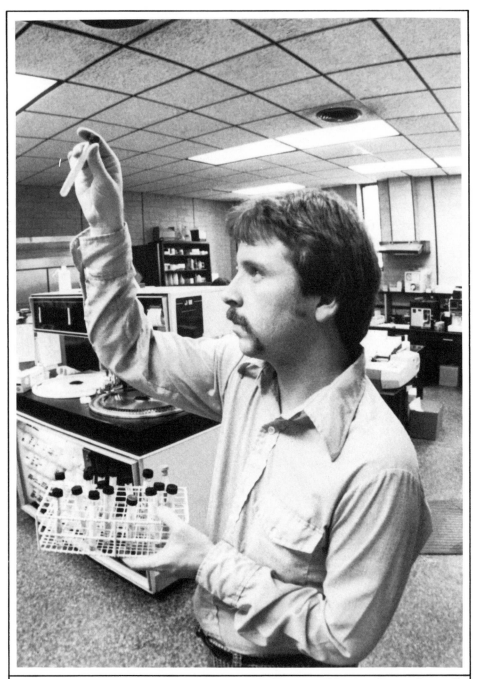

Scientists in the 1980s continue to search for nonaddictive drugs that will bring pain relief without side effects and stimulate the body to produce more of its own pain relievers.

CHAPTER 9

ON THE HORIZON: NEW METHODS OF PAIN RELIEF

Science has come a long way in the search for safe and effective pain relief. Hundreds of drugs in thousands of combinations are available to ease suffering, and pain specialists report that even those people in serious pain can expect enough relief to resume normal activities.

Yet the search continues, particularly for drugs that work as well as narcotics without addictive and sickening side effects and for imaginative new ways to interrupt the transmission of pain signals.

There have been some stunning advances in this area.

Meptazinol, a drug developed by Wyeth Laboratories, for example, activates the body's own opiate-receptor and opiate-release system.

Capsaicin, a substance found in chili pepper, causes nerves to release substance P. Experiments show that although applying capsaicin initially produces a burning pain, continued use produces numbness not unlike a topical anesthetic. The drug holds promise for the relief of joint and muscle pain.

Doctors at the University of Chicago Medical Center are using a new electronic device to alleviate chronic, intractable pain. Electrical current, generated via electrodes planted

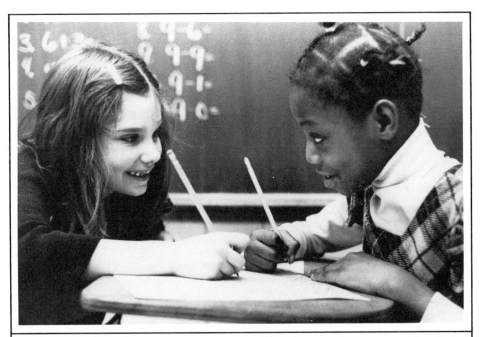

Present and future generations will benefit from studies into pain relief. By the time today's teenagers are raising families, modern "miracle" drugs will be supplanted by even more effective painkillers.

deep in the brain, stimulates the release of endorphins. Patients use a pocket-sized transmitter to send a signal to the electrodes, and pain relief occurs in minutes. This system has already been used in various experiments to treat back pain; in some cases it has completely eliminated the need for narcotics.

Intensive studies are also underway to develop drugs that block bradykinin, the most powerful pain-producing substance yet discovered. Within the past two years, scientists at the University of Colorado Medical Center and elsewhere have identified five bradykinin antagonists that have vast potential against pain from burns, infections, and surgical wounds.

Scientists are developing long-acting narcotics that are effective but do not cause tolerance or addiction.

Thanks to silicon-chip technology, tiny computers joined to even tinier pumps can be implanted in patients with chronic pain to let the patients regulate the administration of narcotics. With safeguards against overdose, these devices promise to eliminate the anxiety and stress of waiting for the next pill or shot and reduce pain in the process.

Stick-on skin patches saturated with slow-release pain medications, such as fentanyl, administer drugs through the skin evenly over long periods of time, enhancing the body's ability to respond to analgesics efficiently.

With chemical and mechanical means, surgeons can permanently damage or cut off pain-nerve pathways and bring long-lasting relief to patients with constant, severe pain. Although these techniques are not without side effects (burning sensations may develop, and the pain may recur within six months), newer microsurgical methods make the procedures safer and far less of a problem than narcotic tolerance and addiction.

In their search for better pain relievers, scientists are using computers to mimic natural molecules and manipulate their chemical makeup. By identifying various types of brain receptors, they can produce synthetic molecules that fit like a key in a lock to receptors that influence pain without influencing or harming other brain and body activities.

At this time, prospects for *the* perfect pain pill are far in the future. But chances are good that by the time contemporary teenagers are raising their own families, some of today's best painkillers will have been made obsolete by safer, more effective drugs.

Until then, teenagers and their families can take comfort in the fact that their access to pain relief is better than at any time in human history.

APPENDIX I

State Agencies for the Prevention and Treatment of Drug Abuse

ALABAMA
Department of Mental Health
Division of Mental Illness and
  Substance Abuse Community
  Programs
200 Interstate Park Drive
P.O. Box 3710
Montgomery, AL 36193
(205) 271-9253

ALASKA
Department of Health and Social
  Services
Office of Alcoholism and Drug
  Abuse
Pouch H-05-F
Juneau, AK 99811
(907) 586-6201

ARIZONA
Department of Health Services
Division of Behavioral Health
  Services
Bureau of Community Services
Alcohol Abuse and Alcoholism
  Section
2500 East Van Buren
Phoenix, AZ 85008
(602) 255-1238

Department of Health Services
Division of Behavioral Health
  Services
Bureau of Community Services
Drug Abuse Section
2500 East Van Buren
Phoenix, AZ 85008
(602) 255-1240

ARKANSAS
Department of Human Services
Office of Alcohol and Drug Abuse
  Prevention
1515 West 7th Avenue
Suite 310
Little Rock, AR 72202
(501) 371-2603

CALIFORNIA
Department of Alcohol and Drug
  Abuse
111 Capitol Mall
Sacramento, CA 95814
(916) 445-1940

COLORADO
Department of Health
Alcohol and Drug Abuse Division
4210 East 11th Avenue
Denver, CO 80220
(303) 320-6137

CONNECTICUT
Alcohol and Drug Abuse
  Commission
999 Asylum Avenue
3rd Floor
Hartford, CT 06105
(203) 566-4145

DELAWARE
Division of Mental Health
Bureau of Alcoholism and Drug
  Abuse
1901 North Dupont Highway
Newcastle, DE 19720
(302) 421-6101

DISTRICT OF COLUMBIA
Department of Human Services
Office of Health Planning and
  Development
601 Indiana Avenue, NW
Suite 500
Washington, D.C. 20004
(202) 724-5641

FLORIDA
Department of Health and
  Rehabilitative Services
Alcoholic Rehabilitation Program
1317 Winewood Boulevard
Room 187A
Tallahassee, FL 32301
(904) 488-0396

Department of Health and
  Rehabilitative Services
Drug Abuse Program
1317 Winewood Boulevard
Building 6, Room 155
Tallahassee, FL 32301
(904) 488-0900

GEORGIA
Department of Human Resources
Division of Mental Health and
  Mental Retardation
Alcohol and Drug Section
618 Ponce De Leon Avenue, NE
Atlanta, GA 30365-2101
(404) 894-4785

HAWAII
Department of Health
Mental Health Division
Alcohol and Drug Abuse Branch
1250 Punch Bowl Street
P.O. Box 3378
Honolulu, HI 96801
(808) 548-4280

IDAHO
Department of Health and Welfare
Bureau of Preventive Medicine
Substance Abuse Section
450 West State
Boise, ID 83720
(208) 334-4368

ILLINOIS
Department of Mental Health and
  Developmental Disabilities
Division of Alcoholism
160 North La Salle Street
Room 1500
Chicago, IL 60601
(312) 793-2907

Illinois Dangerous Drugs
  Commission
300 North State Street
Suite 1500
Chicago, IL 60610
(312) 822-9860

INDIANA
Department of Mental Health
Division of Addiction Services
429 North Pennsylvania Street
Indianapolis, IN 46204
(317) 232-7816

IOWA
Department of Substance Abuse
505 5th Avenue
Insurance Exchange Building
Suite 202
Des Moines, IA 50319
(515) 281-3641

KANSAS
Department of Social Rehabilitation
Alcohol and Drug Abuse Services
2700 West 6th Street
Biddle Building
Topeka, KS 66606
(913) 296-3925

KENTUCKY
Cabinet for Human Resources
Department of Health Services
Substance Abuse Branch
275 East Main Street
Frankfort, KY 40601
(502) 564-2880

LOUISIANA
Department of Health and Human
  Resources
Office of Mental Health and
  Substance Abuse
655 North 5th Street
P.O. Box 4049
Baton Rouge, LA 70821
(504) 342-2565

MAINE
Department of Human Services
Office of Alcoholism and Drug
  Abuse Prevention
Bureau of Rehabilitation
32 Winthrop Street
Augusta, ME 04330
(207) 289-2781

MARYLAND
Alcoholism Control Administration
201 West Preston Street
Fourth Floor
Baltimore, MD 21201
(301) 383-2977

State Health Department
Drug Abuse Administration
201 West Preston Street
Baltimore, MD 21201
(301) 383-3312

MASSACHUSETTS
Department of Public Health
Division of Alcoholism
755 Boylston Street
Sixth Floor
Boston, MA 02116
(617) 727-1960

Department of Public Health
Division of Drug Rehabilitation
600 Washington Street
Boston, MA 02114
(617) 727-8617

MICHIGAN
Department of Public Health
Office of Substance Abuse Services
3500 North Logan Street
P.O. Box 30035
Lansing, MI 48909
(517) 373-8603

MINNESOTA
Department of Public Welfare
Chemical Dependency Program
  Division
Centennial Building
658 Cedar Street
4th Floor
Saint Paul, MN 55155
(612) 296-4614

MISSISSIPPI
Department of Mental Health
Division of Alcohol and Drug Abuse
1102 Robert E. Lee Building
Jackson, MS 39201
(601) 359-1297

MISSOURI
Department of Mental Health
Division of Alcoholism and Drug
  Abuse
2002 Missouri Boulevard
P.O. Box 687
Jefferson City, MO 65102
(314) 751-4942

MONTANA
Department of Institutions
Alcohol and Drug Abuse Division
1539 11th Avenue
Helena, MT 59620
(406) 449-2827

NEBRASKA
Department of Public Institutions
Division of Alcoholism and Drug
Abuse
801 West Van Dorn Street
P.O. Box 94728
Lincoln, NB 68509
(402) 471-2851, Ext. 415

NEVADA
Department of Human Resources
Bureau of Alcohol and Drug Abuse
505 East King Street
Carson City, NV 89710
(702) 885-4790

NEW HAMPSHIRE
Department of Health and Welfare
Office of Alcohol and Drug Abuse
  Prevention
Hazen Drive
Health and Welfare Building
Concord, NH 03301
(603) 271-4627

NEW JERSEY
Department of Health
Division of Alcoholism
129 East Hanover Street CN 362
Trenton, NJ 08625
(609) 292-8949

Department of Health
Division of Narcotic and Drug
  Abuse Control
129 East Hanover Street CN 362
Trenton, NJ 08625
(609) 292-8949

NEW MEXICO
Health and Environment Department
Behavioral Services Division
Substance Abuse Bureau
725 Saint Michaels Drive
P.O. Box 968
Santa Fe, NM 87503
(505) 984-0020, Ext. 304

NEW YORK
Division of Alcoholism and Alcohol
  Abuse
194 Washington Avenue
Albany, NY 12210
(518) 474-5417

Division of Substance Abuse
  Services
Executive Park South
Box 8200
Albany, NY 12203
(518) 457-7629

NORTH CAROLINA
Department of Human Resources
Division of Mental Health, Mental
  Retardation and Substance Abuse
  Services
Alcohol and Drug Abuse Services
325 North Salisbury Street
Albemarle Building
Raleigh, NC 27611
(919) 733-4670

NORTH DAKOTA
Department of Human Services
Division of Alcoholism and Drug
  Abuse
State Capitol Building
Bismarck, ND 58505
(701) 224-2767

OHIO
Department of Health
Division of Alcoholism
246 North High Street
P.O. Box 118
Columbus, OH 43216
(614) 466-3543

Department of Mental Health
Bureau of Drug Abuse
65 South Front Street
Columbus, OH 43215
(614) 466-9023

OKLAHOMA
Department of Mental Health
Alcohol and Drug Programs
4545 North Lincoln Boulevard
Suite 100 East Terrace
P.O. Box 53277
Oklahoma City, OK 73152
(405) 521-0044

OREGON
Department of Human Resources
Mental Health Division
Office of Programs for Alcohol and
   Drug Problems
2575 Bittern Street, NE
Salem, OR 97310
(503) 378-2163

PENNSYLVANIA
Department of Health
Office of Drug and Alcohol
   Programs
Commonwealth and Forster Avenues
Health and Welfare Building
P.O. Box 90
Harrisburg, PA 17108
(717) 787-9857

RHODE ISLAND
Department of Mental Health,
   Mental Retardation and Hospitals
Division of Substance Abuse
Substance Abuse Administration
   Building
Cranston, RI 02920
(401) 464-2091

SOUTH CAROLINA
Commission on Alcohol and Drug
   Abuse
3700 Forest Drive
Columbia, SC 29204
(803) 758-2521

SOUTH DAKOTA
Department of Health
Division of Alcohol and Drug Abuse
523 East Capitol, Joe Foss Building
Pierre, SD 57501
(605) 773-4806

TENNESSEE
Department of Mental Health and
   Mental Retardation
Alcohol and Drug Abuse Services
505 Deaderick Street
James K. Polk Building,
   Fourth Floor
Nashville, TN 37219
(615) 741-1921

TEXAS
Commission on Alcoholism
809 Sam Houston State Office
   Building
Austin, TX 78701
(512) 475-2577
Department of Community Affairs
Drug Abuse Prevention Division
2015 South Interstate Highway 35
P.O. Box 13166
Austin, TX 78711
(512) 443-4100

UTAH
Department of Social Services
Division of Alcoholism and Drugs
150 West North Temple
Suite 350
P.O. Box 2500
Salt Lake City, UT 84110
(801) 533-6532

VERMONT
Agency of Human Services
Department of Social and
   Rehabilitation Services
Alcohol and Drug Abuse Division
103 South Main Street
Waterbury, VT 05676
(802) 241-2170

VIRGINIA
Department of Mental Health and
  Mental Retardation
Division of Substance Abuse
109 Governor Street
P.O. Box 1797
Richmond, VA 23214
(804) 786-5313

WASHINGTON
Department of Social and Health
  Service
Bureau of Alcohol and Substance
  Abuse
Office Building—44 W
Olympia, WA 98504
(206) 753-5866

WEST VIRGINIA
Department of Health
Office of Behavioral Health Services
Division on Alcoholism and Drug
  Abuse
1800 Washington Street East
Building 3 Room 451
Charleston, WV 25305
(304) 348-2276

WISCONSIN
Department of Health and Social
  Services
Division of Community Services
Bureau of Community Programs
Alcohol and Other Drug Abuse
  Program Office
1 West Wilson Street
P.O. Box /851
Madison, WI 53707
(608) 266-2717

WYOMING
Alcohol and Drug Abuse Programs
Hathaway Building
Cheyenne, WY 82002
(307) 777-7115, Ext. 7118

GUAM
Mental Health & Substance Abuse
  Agency
P.O. Box 20999
Guam 96921

PUERTO RICO
Department of Addiction Control
  Services
Alcohol Abuse Programs
P.O. Box B-Y Rio Piedras Station
Rio Piedras, PR 00928
(809) 763-5014

Department of Addiction Control
  Services
Drug Abuse Programs
P.O. Box B-Y Rio Piedras Station
Rio Piedras, PR 00928
(809) 764-8140

VIRGIN ISLANDS
Division of Mental Health,
  Alcoholism & Drug Dependency
  Services
P.O. Box 7329
Saint Thomas, Virgin Islands 00801
(809) 774-7265

AMERICAN SAMOA
LBJ Tropical Medical Center
Department of Mental Health Clinic
Pago Pago, American Samoa 96799

TRUST TERRITORIES
Director of Health Services
Office of the High Commissioner
Saipan, Trust Territories 96950

APPENDIX II

A Selected List
of Pain Relievers

Physicians and pharmacists are the best sources of information about prescription and nonprescription drugs and their side effects and actions.

The following list is not comprehensive, but meant only as a guide to some categories of pain-relieving drugs that teenagers are likely to hear about. Brand names are capitalized.

Some tips for using ANY pain reliever:

■ NEVER use another person's prescription medication.

■ READ labels carefully for indications (what the drug is legally approved for), dosage (how much to take, when, and how often), contraindications (who should not take them), and side effects.

■ FOLLOW instructions on dosage carefully. More is not necessarily better and may hurt you. Less is not necessarily safer and may do you no good.

■ DON'T combine drugs without an OK from your physician or pharmacist. Even over-the-counter medications, when taken together, may produce dangerous interactions that are not a problem if the drugs are taken alone.

■ STOP taking any drug that produces pain, dizziness, serious nausea, confusion, or other serious symptoms. Stop immediately and TELL someone about them.

■ AVOID all drugs if you are pregnant or think you might be. Talk to a physician before using any medication, prescription or nonprescription.

■ BUY only approved drugs in reputable retail outlets. Approved drugs may be sold by brand name or generic name. Generic drugs are often less expensive and sold under the name of the supermarket or pharmacy that sells them. A brand name is a copyrighted trade name under which a drug is sold. The generic name is the chemical name of the drug. For example, Tylenol is the McNeil Laboratories brand of acetaminophen, and acetaminophen is the generic name.

Prescription Analgesics

NAME: Darvon (Eli Lilly)
GENERIC NAME/ACTIVE INGREDIENT:
    propoxyphene hydrochloride
CATEGORY: mild narcotic
FORM: capsule
USES: mild to moderate pain
SIDE EFFECTS: dizziness, sedation, nausea, vomiting, constipation, rashes, headache, weakness, euphoria, potential for abuse and dependency

NAME: Demerol (Winthrop)
GENERIC NAME/ACTIVE INGREDIENT:
    meperidene hydrochloride
CATEGORY: narcotic
FORM: tablet, liquid
USES: moderate to severe pain
SIDE EFFECTS: same as Darvon, but far more likely to be habit-forming

NAME: Dilaudid (Knoll)
GENERIC NAME/ACTIVE INGREDIENT:
    hydromorphone hydrochloride
CATEGORY: narcotic
FORM: injectable, tablet
USES: moderate to severe pain
SIDE EFFECTS: same as Demerol

NAME: Empirin with Codeine (Burroughs Wellcome)
GENERIC NAME/ACTIVE INGREDIENT:
    aspirin, codeine phosphate
CATEGORY: mild narcotic
FORM: tablets
USES: mild to moderate pain in normal dosages

SIDE EFFECTS: similar to Darvon

NAME: Fiorinal (Sandoz)
GENERIC NAME/ACTIVE INGREDIENT:
    butalbitol, aspirin, caffeine
CATEGORY: barbiturate sedative, analgesic
FORM: capsules, tablets
USES: mild to moderate pain accompanied by tension or anxiety
SIDE EFFECTS: drowsiness, nausea, constipation, dizziness, and rashes, potential to be habit-forming.

NAME: Motrin (Upjohn)
GENERIC NAME/ACTIVE INGREDIENT:
    ibuprofen
CATEGORY: nonsteroidal anti-inflammatory analgesic
FORM: tablets
USES: mild to moderate pain, menstrual and premenstrual cramps
SIDE EFFECTS: nausea, chest pain, heartburn, digestive upset, gas, dizziness, headache, insomnia, decreased appetite, depression, fever

NAME: Percodan (DuPont)
GENERIC NAME/ACTIVE INGREDIENT:
    oxycodone hydrochloride, oxycodone terephthalate, aspirin
CATEGORY: narcotic
FORM: tablets

USES: moderate to moderately severe pain
SIDE EFFECTS: same as Demerol

NAME: Talwin Tablets (Winthrop-Breon)
GENERIC NAME/ACTIVE INGREDIENT: pentazocine hydrochloride, aspirin
CATEGORY: synthetic narcotic
FORM: tablets
USES: moderate pain
SIDE EFFECTS: same as narcotics, but

also blurred vision, hallucinations, tremors

NAME: Tylenol with Codeine (McNeil)
GENERIC NAME/ACTIVE INGREDIENT: codeine phosphate, acetaminophen
CATEGORY: mild narcotic
FORM: tablets
USES: mild to moderately severe pain
SIDE EFFECTS: drowsiness, constipation, nausea

Non-Prescription Analgesics

NAME: Advil (Whitehall)
GENERIC NAME/ACTIVE INGREDIENT: ibuprofen
CATEGORY: nonsteroidal anti-inflammatory analgesic
FORM: tablets
USES: fever and mild to moderate pain
SIDE EFFECTS: heartburn, upset stomach; in people allergic to aspirin, asthma, swelling, hives, shock

NAME: Alka-Seltzer (Miles)
GENERIC NAME/ACTIVE INGREDIENT: buffered aspirin, sodium bicarbonate, citric acid
CATEGORY: analgesic, antacid
FORM: effervescent tablets
USES: headache, upset stomach, "hangovers"
SIDE EFFECTS: allergic reactions in sensitive individuals, bleeding, stomach upset, nausea, bloat-

ing; aspirin products should not be used by teenagers with flu or chicken pox

NAME: Aspergum (Plough)
GENERIC NAME/ACTIVE INGREDIENT: aspirin
CATEGORY: analgesic
FORM: coated gum
USES: sore throat and mouth pain
SIDE EFFECTS: same as aspirin

NAME: Bayer Aspirin (Glenbrook)
GENERIC NAME/ACTIVE INGREDIENT: acetylsalicylic acid
CATEGORY: analgesic
FORM: tablets
USES: fever, swelling, mild to moderate headaches and pain associated with colds, flu, arthritis, dental work, menstruation
SIDE EFFECTS: allergic reactions in sensitive individuals, bleeding,

stomach upset, nausea, bloating; aspirin products should not be used by teenagers with flu or chicken pox

NAME: Ben Gay (Leeming)
GENERIC NAME/ACTIVE INGREDIENT: methyl salicylate (oil of wintergreen), menthol
CATEGORY: counterirritant (reddens the skin and warms it)
FORMS: ointment
USES: muscle aches and pains
SIDE EFFECTS: poisonous if ingested

NAME: Bromo-Seltzer (Warner-Lambert)
GENERIC NAME/ACTIVE INGREDIENT: acetaminophen, sodium bicarbonate, citric acid
CATEGORY: analgesic, antacid
FORM: effervescent tablets
USES: same as Alka-Seltzer
SIDE EFFECTS: in overdoses, possible liver damage

NAME: Bufferin (Bristol-Myers)
GENERIC NAME/ACTIVE INGREDIENT: aspirin, magnesium carbonate, aluminum glycinate
CATEGORY: analgesic
FORM: tablets
USES: same as aspirin, acetaminophen; added ingredients buffer the aspirin, reducing stomach irritation
SIDE EFFECTS: same as aspirin

NAME: Coricidin (Schering)
GENERIC NAME/ACTIVE INGREDIENT: aspirin, chlorpheniramine maleate

CATEGORY: analgesic, antihistamine
FORM: tablets
USES: colds, flu with fever, pain, congestion
SIDE EFFECTS: same as aspirin, drowsiness

NAME: Cortaid (Upjohn)
GENERIC NAME/ACTIVE INGREDIENT: hydrocortisone
CATEGORY: steroidal anti-inflammatory
FORM: ointment, cream
USES: relieves mild pain and itching on skin
SIDE EFFECTS: occasional allergic reaction and irritation of skin

NAME: Datril (Bristol-Myers)
GENERIC NAME/ACTIVE INGREDIENT: acetaminophen
CATEGORY: analgesic
FORM: tablets
USES: pain, fever, inflammation; same as aspirin
SIDE EFFECTS in overdoses, possible liver damage

NAME: Dermoplast (Ayerst)
GENERIC NAME/ACTIVE INGREDIENT: benzocaine, menthol
CATEGORY: topical anesthetic
FORM: spray
USES: skin itches and pain
SIDE EFFECTS: in a very small percentage of users, local skin irritation

NAME: Dristan (Whitehall)
GENERIC NAME/ACTIVE INGREDIENT: phenylephrine hydrochloride, chlorpheniramine maleate,

acetaminophen, caffeine
CATEGORY: analgesic, decongestant, antihistamine
FORM: tablets
USES: mild to moderate pain, fever, congestion
SIDE EFFECTS: same as acetaminophen, drowsiness, irritability, dizziness, insomnia.

NAME: Excedrin (Bristol-Myers)
GENERIC NAME/ACTIVE INGREDIENT: aspirin, acetaminophen, caffeine
CATEGORY: analgesic
FORM: tablets
USES: mild to moderate pain, fever
SIDE EFFECTS: same as aspirin, acetaminophen; caffeine may produce insomnia, irritability

NAME: Listerine Antiseptic Lozenges (Warner-Lambert)
GENERIC NAME/ACTIVE INGREDIENT: hexylresorcinol
CATEGORY: topical anesthetic
FORM: lozenges
USES: sore throat and mouth pain
SIDE EFFECTS: rare reports of allergic reactions

NAME: Nupercainal (CIBA)
GENERIC NAME/ACTIVE INGREDIENT: dibucaine
CATEGORY: topical anesthetic
FORM: cream, suppositories
USES: hemorrhoid and other ano-rectal pain and itching
SIDE EFFECTS: rare allergic reactions

APPENDIX III

Key to Pronunciation

acetaminophen (aah-CEE-tah-MIN-o-fen)

acetylcholine (AAH-se-teal-KO-lean)

bradykinin (BRAY-dee-KIE-nin)

dopamine (DO-pa-mean)

enkephalins (en-KEF-ah-lins)

ibuprofen (EYE-bew-PRO-fen)

norepinephrine (NOR-eh-pin-EH-frin)

prostaglandins (PROSS-ta-GLAN-dins)

APPENDIX IV

Sample Pain Diary

If you are experiencing any sort of long-term pain, keeping track of it in this sample pain diary will help you to assess your own condition. And, just as importantly, it will provide your family doctor with accurate information.

DAY	TIME	LOCATION OF PAIN	TYPE OF PAIN	SEVERITY*	ACTIVITY**
2/22	1 p.m.	all across lower back	sharp ache	moderate	sitting on an airplane
2/23	3 a.m.	all across lower back; spreading down left leg	sharp ache; throbbing	severe	awakened from sleep; up the rest of the night; barely able to get out of bed
2/23	all day	pain continues but gradually diminishes to dull ache			great difficulty sitting down and standing up
2/24	all day	pain no longer in leg; in back only	dull ache	mild	less difficulty in moving
2/25	a.m. c̄ p.m.	same pain, but less intense	dull ache	mild	hurts only after prolonged sitting; walking and gentle stretching seems to help
3/26	at work	only in small of back	dull ache	mild	sitting; no real trouble moving around anymore

*Mild, Moderate, Severe
**What subject was doing at the time the pain was noticed, activities just preceding the onset of pain, mood, worries, etc.

Further Reading

American Society of Hospital Pharmacists. *Consumer Drug Digest.* New York: Facts on File, 1982.

Jones, Judith K. *Good Housekeeping Guide to Medicines and Drugs Yearbook.* New York: The Hearst Corporation, 1977.

Knight, Nancy. *Pain and its Relief: An Exhibition at the National Museum of American History.* Washington, D.C.: Smithsonian Institution, 1983.

Physicians Desk Reference 1986. Oradell, New Jersey: Medical Economics Company, Inc., 1986.

Stern, Edward L. *Prescription Drugs and Their Side Effects. 4th Edition.* New York: Perigee Books, 1983.

Zimmerman, David R. *The Essential Guide to Nonprescription Drugs.* New York: Harper and Row, 1983.

Glossary

acetylcholine a neurotransmitter found throughout the body that is believed to play an important role in the transmission of nerve impulses, especially at synapses; its actions at nicotinic receptors is mimicked by nicotine

acetylsalicylic acid a white crystalline solid formed when acetic anhydride interacts with salicylic acid. This compound is used as an analgesic

acute a condition in which the symptoms are often severe but of short duration

addiction a condition caused by repeated drug use, characterized by a compulsive urge to continue using the drug, a tendency to increase the dosage, and physiological and/or psychological dependence

adjuvant a drug added to another prescription drug to speed up or intensify its actions

agonist a muscle that contracts

alkaloids one of many organic substances that contain nitrogen and strongly affect body functions; drugs such as morphine and cocaine are alkaloids

analgesic any of a number of drugs that relieve pain

anesthetic any one of a number of drugs that produce a loss of partial or total sensation in a bodily organ while the individual retains consciousness

antagonist a muscle or drug that counteracts the action of another muscle or drug

autonomic nervous system the part of the nervous system that is concerned with control of involuntary bodily functions

benign a condition that only appears once and does not develop into something more serious

biofeedback a training program in which an individual learns to control his autonomic nervous system

bradykinin a polypeptide (two or more amino acids) that is capable of considerable biological activity and is composed of plasma

central nervous system consisting of the brain, spinal cord, and connecting nerves

chronic referring to a condition or disease that arises and does not appreciably change over a long period of time

dolorogenic causing pain

dopamine a neurotransmitter that is synthesized by the adrenal gland

epinephrine a hormone secreted by the adrenal medulla in response to splanchic stimulation (stimulation of the viscera or organs within a body cavity)

ergotamine a crystalline alkaloid derived from the fungus *Claviceps purpurea*, which grows on rye

freebasing a potent and dangerous method whereby street cocaine is mixed with ammonium hydroxide and heated, then smoked in a pipe for a quick and addictive high

intravenous within or into a vein

morphine a main alkaloid in opium that is often used as an analgesic/sedative

narcotic a drug that relieves pain and produces sleep in small doses, but causes stupors and unconsciousness in larger amounts; examples of these drugs are opium, codeine, morphine, and heroin

neurotransmitter a chemical released by neurons that transmits nerve impulses across a synapse

nociception a nerve center's perception of painful stimuli

norepinephrine a neurotransmitter found in the autonomic nervous system; chemically, norepinephrine is a catecholamine (biologically active amine)

nostrum a secret or "quack" (ineffective) remedy

opiates compounds from the milky juice of the poppy plant *Papaver somniferum*, including opium, morphine, codeine, and heroin

panacea a cure-all, a remedy

peptide a compound containing two or more amino acids

physical dependence adaption of the body to the presence of a drug such that its absence produces withdrawal symptoms

placebo an inactive substance used for control groups in drug experiments or to placate a patient

prostaglandins a group of fatty acid derivatives present in many body tissues

psychological dependence a condition in which the drug user craves a drug to maintain a sense of well-being and feels discomfort when deprived of it

psychosomatic an illness that is caused or aggravated by the emotional or mental state of the patient

receptor a specialized component of a cell that combines with a chemical substance to alter the function of a cell; for example, nerve cell receptors combine with neurotransmitters

referred pain pain felt in an area outside of the point of origin

reticular formation a group of cells and fibers connecting the motor and sensory nerves to the brain stem

Reyes syndrome an illness identified in children under 18 years old that follows viral infections; it is characterized by acute brain dysfunctions and fatty infiltration of the liver or other organs

soporific producing sleep

synapse the narrow gap between neurons; the point at which a nerve impulse is transmitted from one neuron to another

thalamus the part of the brain that receives pain messages and then relays them to other parts of the brain

tolerance a decrease of susceptibility to the effects of a drug due to its continued administration, resulting in the user's need to increase the drug dosage in order to achieve the effects experienced previously

topical pertinent to a definite local area

withdrawal the physiological and psychological effects of discontinued use of a drug

Picture Credits

Index

Joann Ellison Rodgers, M.S. (Columbia), became Deputy Director of Public Affairs and Director of Media Relations for the Johns Hopkins Medical Institutions in Baltimore, Maryland, in 1984 after 18 years as an award-winning science journalist and widely read columnist for the Hearst newspapers.

Solomon H. Snyder, M.D. is Distinguished Service Professor of Neuroscience, Pharmacology and Psychiatry at The Johns Hopkins University School of Medicine. He has served as president of the Society for Neuroscience and in 1978 received the Albert Lasker Award in Medical Research. He has authored *Uses of Marijuana, Madness and the Brain, The Troubled Mind, Biological Aspects of Mental Disorder,* and edited *Perspective in Neuropharmacology: A Tribute to Julius Axelrod.* Professor Snyder was a research associate with Dr. Axelrod at the National Institutes of Health.

Barry L. Jacobs, Ph.D., is currently a professor in the program of neuroscience at Princeton University. Professor Jacobs is author of *Serotonin Neurotransmission and Behavior* and *Hallucinogens: Neurochemical, Behavioral and Clinical Perspectives.* He has written many journal articles in the field of neuroscience and contributed numerous chapters to books on behavior and brain science. He has been a member of several panels of the National Institute of Mental Health.

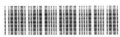